# ERCP in Pediatric Practice: Diagnosis and Treatment

# ERCP in Pediatric Practice: Diagnosis and Treatment

**Moises Guelrud**
*Chief Gastroenterology Department, Hospital General del Oeste,
Ministerio de Sanidad y Asistencia Social,
Los Magallanes, Caracas, Venezuela*

**David L. Carr-Locke**
*Director of Endoscopy, Division of Gastroenterology,
Brigham and Women's Hospital, 75 Francis Street,
Boston MA 02115, USA*

**Victor L. Fox**
*Director of Endoscopy, Division of Gastroenterology, Children's Hospital,
Instructor of Pediatrics, Harvard Medical School,
300 Longwood Avenue, Boston MA 02115, USA*


I S I S
MEDICAL
MEDIA

Oxford

© 1997 by Isis Medical Media Ltd.
58 St Aldates
Oxford OX1 1ST, UK


First published 1997




British Library Cataloguing in Publication Data.
A catalogue record for this title is available from
the British Library.

ISBN 1 899066 05 5

Guelrud, M (Moises)
ERCP in Pediatric Practice: Diagnosis and Treatment
Moises Guelrud, David L. Carr-Locke, Victor L. Fox


Always refer to the manufacturer's Prescribing
Information before prescribing drugs cited in this book.


**Typeset by**
Marksbury Multimedia Ltd., Midsomer Norton, Avon, UK

**Printed and bound by**
Printek S.A.L., Bilbao, Spain

**Distributed in the U.S.A. by**
Mosby-Year Book, Inc.
11830 Westline Industrial Drive
St. Louis, MO 63146, USA

**Distributed in the rest of the world by**
Oxford University Press
Saxon Way West
Corby, Northamptonshire, NN18 9ES, UK

# Contents

# Foreword

Endoscopic retrograde cholangiopancreatography (ERCP) was first described almost thirty years ago in the adult population. Initial reports of successful ERCP in isolated pediatric patients were published a few years later. Development of pediatric duodenoscopes, expansion of the indications and an increasing number of trained endoscopists led to a greater number of procedures being performed in children. Interventional endoscopic procedures initially performed in adult patients have also been adapted to smaller patients. Endoscopic sphincterotomy, pancreatic and common duct stone extraction, drainage of pancreatic pseudocysts and placement of prostheses have all been performed in children with success rates similar to those in the adult population.

Drs Guelrud, Carr-Locke and Fox, all experts in the field, have written a comprehensive text drawing from their own experience and those of others who have pioneered the development of ERCP in children. The authors initiate the discussion with a thorough review of the technique of ERCP in children including instrumentation, indications and potential complications. The book is subsequently divided into two major sections, focusing on diseases of the hepatobiliary system and pancreas. The authors have thoughtfully described the diseases and the potential role of ERCP in diagnosis and management. The text is liberally illustrated with clear radiographs and supplemented with line drawings. The authors make a strong case for increasing the use of ERCP in the evaluation of infants with neonatal jaundice and in the management of children with recurrent pancreatitis.

My congratulations to Drs Guelrud, Carr-Locke and Fox on the success of their efforts. Routine visualization of the pancreatic and biliary duct in infants and children in the last decade has substantially influenced the diagnosis and treatment of pancreatobiliary disease. The publication of a monograph on ERCP in children represents a milestone in the acceptance of the procedure in young patients. The book will become a standard in the field and be a valuable reference to physicians participating in the care of children with pancreatic and biliary disorders.

Robert Wyllie M.D.
Chairman, Department of Subspecialty Pediatrics,
Head, Section of Pediatric Gastroenterology
Cleveland Clinic Foundation, 9500 Euclid Ave., Cleveland, Ohio 44195, USA

# Preface

In the past two decades, visualization of the biliary tree and the pancreatic duct by the use of endoscopic retrograde cholangiopancreatography (ERCP) has substantially influenced the evaluation and treatment of patients with suspected pancreatic and biliary disease. The first endoscopic cannulation of the ampulla of Vater was described by McCune and colleagues in 1968 using a gastroscope. Since then, ERCP has undergone several important technical developments with lateral viewing endoscopes becoming available for adults in 1970, and smaller duodenoscopes with appropriate accessories available for neonates and infants since 1983. Since then, a burgeoning literature has followed describing new endoscopic approaches to management of pancreatic and biliary diseases including therapeutic applications in children.

These procedures require an endoscopy team skilled in duodenoscopy and the successful performance of radiographic examination of the biliary tree and pancreatic duct. Hence, the endoscopist must be already well-trained in the use of forward-viewing upper gastrointestinal endoscopes. The first reports of ERCP in infants and children were chiefly from adult gastroenterologists experienced with such techniques. The growth in number and availability of skilled endoscopists has resulted in more frequent performance of ERCP in children. Moreover, the acquired ability to perform therapeutic endoscopic procedures is also applicable to children and adolescents. Techniques such as endoscopic sphincterotomy, biliary drainage, extraction of common bile duct and pancreatic duct stones, implantation of endoprostheses, and drainage of pancreatic pseudocysts are beginning to be used in children with an overall success rate similar to that reported for adult patients. However, these procedures are generally performed in a tertiary care facility by endoscopists who maintain a high volume of such activity.

This book reflects 12 years of experience with ERCP in children. Our aims are to assist in the training of pediatric gastroenterologists, to make ERCP findings in children more familiar to pediatricians, as well as radiologists, surgeons, and gastroenterologists interested in children, to provide a stimulus to those endoscopists who perform ERCP but whose experience and training has been limited to adults, and to extend the application of diagnostic and therapeutic endoscopy in a pediatric setting.

M. Guelrud
D. L. Carr-Locke
V. L. Fox

# Acknowledgments

We are most grateful to Dr Domingo Jaen, Chief of the Pediatric Gastrointestinal Unit at Hospital General del Oeste, since most of the material upon which this book is based was collected from his patients. We want to give special thanks to the Pediatric Gastroenterology fellows; without their help this book could not have been produced. We would also like to thank Dr Sonia Mendoza for her genuine concern and help through the years. We are also grateful to the many pediatric gastroenterologists in Venezuela, and especially to Dr Hans Romer and Dr Pedro Torres from the Gastroenterology Department at Hospital de Niños J.M. de los Rios in Caracas, who provided us with their patients.

We also wish to thank Mr Oswaldo Velasquez for the preparation of all the photographic material used in this book.

Finally, we wish to give special thanks to Mrs Raiza Espinoza, for her efficient assistance in typing and expediting the preparation of the manuscript.

**To Mary, Daniel, Andres and Max**
in appreciation of their patience and encouragement

# CHAPTER 1

# Technique

## Patient preparation, sedation and anesthesia

While there is growing experience with ERCP among pediatric gastroenterologists, few have sufficient volume to ensure solo competence with complicated or therapeutic ERCP. The pediatric gastroenterologist does, however, have expertise in the indications for ERCP in children and in sedation of children undergoing endoscopic procedures as well as the overall medical management of pediatric patients. A close working collaboration between an adult and a pediatric gastroenterologist is, therefore, important during both patient preparation and the procedure itself.

The preparation and sedation of a child undergoing ERCP is similar to that used for upper gastrointestinal endoscopy. The procedure should be explained to the child in a manner appropriate for the age and level of intellectual and emotional development. Sedation and analgesia are often major concerns of the child and the parents. Details about the effects and risks of various medications and anesthesia options should be shared. The potential risks and benefits of the procedure should be carefully explained and written informed consent should be obtained from the parents or guardian. Additional comfort and security is provided by encouraging children to bring transition objects (e.g. stuffed animals, blankets) and by asking parents to remain with the child during initiation of sedation.

Before choosing the type of sedation, the endoscopist must determine the anesthesia risk category of the patient. This should take into account the presence and severity of coexisting systemic disease, placing particular emphasis on cardiac, respiratory, and neurologic dysfunction. A scale of increasing risk (I–V) used by the American Society of Anesthesiologists (see Table 1.1) is suitable for this purpose.

***Table 1.1*** American Society of Anesthesiologists physical status classification

| | |
|---|---|
| Class I | A normally healthy patient |
| Class II | A patient with mild systemic disease |
| Class III | A patient with severe systemic disease |
| Class IV | A patient with severe systemic disease that is a constant threat to life |
| Class V | A moribund patient who is not expected to survive without the operation |

Reproduced by permission of PEDIATRICS Vol 89, Pages 1110–1115, Copyright 1992.

Patients classified as ASA I–II (and selected ASA III) are generally considered safe candidates for intravenous conscious sedation. Higher risk category patients should receive general anesthesia with endotracheal intubation. Additional considerations include: (1) the size of the endoscope relative to the size of the child, i.e. potential airway compression, (2) anticipation of painful, prolonged or technically difficult procedures, (3) a history of previous unsatisfactory sedation, and (4) major behavioral disorders.

Since young children and some adolescents are unable to fully cooperate with procedures under conscious sedation, a state of deep sedation from which the patient is not easily aroused is often required. Patients are at risk of partial or complete loss of protective reflexes in such a deeply sedated state and, therefore, require extremely vigilant monitoring and immediate access to resuscitative support. Prone positioning on a fluoroscopic imaging table further complicates airway management for a patient who becomes unstable. General anesthesia with endotracheal intubation offers superior control over sedation and respiratory support. The endoscopist must choose between conscious sedation and general anesthesia after considering the above risks and taking into account personal skill and experience, expected complexity of the procedure, and lastly, cost.

The American Academy of Pediatrics, Committee on Drugs, has established guidelines for appropriate monitoring of children undergoing conscious sedation (1). One assistant, generally a nurse who has training and experience in airway management, should continuously monitor the patient's vital signs and respiratory effort, administer additional medication as needed, and not share other duties during the procedure. A second endoscopy assistant is required to assist with equipment.

Essential monitoring equipment includes a pulse oxymeter, an ECG monitor and a blood pressure cuff preferably attached to an automated monitor. Vacuum suction and a continuous source of pressurized 100% oxygen are also required. Resuscitation equipment should include an anesthesia bag with several sizes of masks, medications and equipment for airway intubation, and a defibrillator.

Vital signs must be documented prior to the administration of medications. Heart rate and oxygen saturation must be continuously monitored during the procedure. The child's head position and restraining devices must be frequently checked to ensure airway patency. There must be careful documentation of the route, time and dose of all administered medications. Transient oxygen desaturation is common during pediatric endoscopy. Routine supplemental oxygen given via nasal cannula or blow-by mask prevents or corrects this desaturation in most cases.

A pre-sedation fasting period is required for all patients to avoid aspiration of gastric contents. Since motility and diet (for infants) differ between children and adults, the fasting period or dietary precautions for children are age-dependent (see Table 1.2).

Most children can be adequately sedated with a combination of meperidine (2–4 mg/kg, maximum 100 mg) and diazepam (0.1–0.3 mg/kg, maximum 15 mg) or midazolam (0.1–0.3 mg/kg, maximum 15 mg). Fentanyl (1–4 μg/kg, maximum 100 μg), a highly potent and short-acting opioid, may be substituted for meperidine. To obtain adequate sedation, children frequently require much higher doses of midazolam on a milligram per kilogram basis than adults. These medications should be titrated by giving incremental doses every 3–5 minutes while continuously assessing respiratory effort, oxygen saturation and cardiovascular status until the desired depth of sedation is reached. While some endoscopists feel that neonates do not require sedation, others disagree. Neonates certainly respond to the stress of noxious or painful stimuli. Their response is less overtly apparent and, therefore, more easily overlooked or ignored. Routine use of topical analgesia of the pharynx in neonates and young infants is similarly controversial. Benzocaine (10%) paste

**Table 1.2**  Dietary precautions for elective sedation

**Infants less than 6 months old**

no milk or solids for 4 hours prior to scheduled procedure

**Infants and children 6–36 months**

no milk or solids for 6 hours prior to scheduled procedure

**Children older than 36 months**

no milk or solids for 8 hours prior to scheduled procedure

**All ages**

clear liquids may continue until 2 hours prior to scheduled procedure and include:

water, oral electrolyte solutions, clear juices, non-carbonated beverages, and popsicles

solid food includes:

candy, chewing gum, non-liquid milk products, and any juice with pulp

Reproduced from Walker W.A. *et al.* Pediatric Gastrointestinal Disease: Pathophysiology, Diagnosis, Management. 2nd Edition, 1996. With permission from Mosby-Year Book Inc., St. Louis.

can be applied to the pharynx of an infant with a finger or soft-tipped applicator. Large doses of topical xylocaine should be avoided in infants given the potential for systemic toxicity. In general, children receiving deep sedation derive less benefit from topical analgesia than those receiving lighter or conscious sedation.

Post-procedure monitoring is the same as for other endoscopic procedures requiring sedation. Vital signs are monitored and recorded until the child meets appropriate criteria for discharge, usually within a period of 2–4 hours. Families should be alerted to the signs of post-ERCP pancreatitis which typically arises within 12–24 hours. Persistent pain, fever, bleeding or other problems should be reported immediately. While children can often be sent home the same day of the procedure, overnight observation in hospital or within close proximity of the hospital is recommended for higher risk patients and procedures and for patients who must travel a long distance to return home.

There are no pediatric data to guide antibiotic prophylaxis for ERCP. Prophylactic antibiotics should be used to prevent endocarditis in susceptible patients in the same manner as upper gastrointestinal endoscopy. Patients at greatest risk are those with prosthetic heart valves, a previous history of endocarditis, or surgically constructed systemic-pulmonary shunts or conduits (see Tables 1.3 and 1.4). While the incidence of bacteremia during ERCP is low, patients who are organ transplant recipients or are otherwise immunocompromised and patients with indwelling catheters should be given individual consideration for antibiotic prophylaxis. Finally, patients with cystic or obstructing lesions of the biliary or pancreatic ducts should be given antibiotic prophylaxis to prevent cholangitis or infective pancreatitis.

Additional medications which may be useful during ERCP include glucagon and buscopan (hyoscine-N-butyl bromide) to reduce duodenal motility, and secretin to facilitate identification and cannulation of the minor papilla.

## Instruments

In neonates and infants younger than 12 months, ERCP is performed with a special Olympus pediatric duodenoscope (PJF; Olympus Corporation of America, Lake Success, NY) (3). The lateral view instrument (Fig. 1.1) is 1310 mm in total length, with a working length of 1130 mm. The insertion tube diameter is 8.5 mm with a distal tip of 8.8 mm. This fixed focus

**Table 1.3**  Endocarditis prophylaxis

---

*Endocarditis prophylaxis recommended*
Prosthetic cardiac valves, including bioprosthetic and homograft valves
Previous bacterial endocarditis, even in the absence of heart disease
Most congenital cardiac malformations
Rheumatic and other acquired valvular dysfunction, even after valvular surgery
Hypertrophic cardiomyopathy
Mitral valve prolapse with valvular regurgitation

*Endocarditis prophylaxis not recommended*
Isolated secundum atrial septal defect
Surgical repair without residua beyond 6 months of secundum atrial septal defect, ventricular septal defect, or
    patent ductus arteriosus
Previous coronary artery bypass graft surgery
Mitral valve prolapse without valvular regurgitation
Physiologic, functional or innocent heart murmurs
Previous Kawasaki disease without valvular dysfunction
Previous rheumatic fever without valvular dysfunction
Cardiac pacemakers and implanted defibrillators

---

Reproduced from Dajani *et al.* Prevention of bacterial endocarditis: recommendations by the American Heart Association, JAMA 264: 2919–2922, 1990; American Medical Association with permission.

adjustment endoscope has a field view of 80°, an observation range between 5 and 60 mm, an upward bending capability of 120°, and a right, left and downward bending capability of 90°. The length of the bending tip is 53 mm. The forceps channel is 2 mm in diameter and has an elevator on its tip.

A thinner prototype Olympus duodenoscope with an insertion tube diameter of 7.5 mm has been manufactured without a cannula elevator. The authors evaluating this instrument found no difference in their ability for selective cannulation with this new instrument as compared with the PJF duodenoscope and concluded that the cannula elevator appears not

**Table 1.4**  Drug regimens for endocarditis prophylaxis

---

*Standard regimen*
Ampicillin 50 mg/kg (max. 2.0 g) and gentamicin 2.0 mg/kg—adult 1.5 mg/kg—(max. 80 mg) IV or IM 30 minutes before procedure; followed by amoxicillin 50 mg/kg (max. 1.5 g) orally 6 hours after initial dose; or repeat parenteral regimen 8 hours after the initial dose

*Ampicillin/amoxicillin/penicillin-allergic patient regimen*
Intravenous administration of vancomycin 20 mg/kg (max. 1.0 g) over 1 hour plus gentamicin 2.0 mg/kg—adult 1.5 mg/kg—(max. 80 mg) IV or IM, 1 hour before procedure; may be repeated once 8 hours after initial dose

*Low risk patient regimen*
Amoxicillin 50 mg/kg (max. 3.0 g) orally 1 hour before procedure; then 25 mg/kg (max. 1.5 g) 6 hours after initial dose

---

Reproduced from Dajani *et al.* Prevention of bacterial endocarditis: recommendations by the American Heart Association, JAMA 264: 2919–2922, 1990; American Medical Association with permission.

to be needed (4). We (MG personal experience) tested the instrument in 11 young infants and failed to cannulate the papilla of Vater in two patients younger than 49 days. The procedure was repeated with the PJF instrument and the papilla was cannulated in both patients. We found that in some patients maneuvering the tip of the instrument is not enough to bring the papilla en face. The newest Olympus pediatric duodenoscope (PJF 7.5), which has an insertion tube diameter of 7.5 mm, a channel of 2.0 mm, and an elevator, has recently become commercially available (Fig. 1.2). This is currently the preferred instrument for infants. The use of a pediatric duodenoscope is mandatory in neonates and in infants younger than 12 months and is preferred for children younger than 3 years. A standard adult duodenoscope (insertion tube diameter approximately 11 mm) can be used for older children and adolescents.

Pediatric duodenoscopes with a 2.0 mm channel will permit passage of catheters and sphincterotomes up to 5 FR diameter. Custom ordered 3 FR catheters are more maneuverable in a 2.0 mm channel endoscope, although they are quite delicate and crimp easily. More complicated therapeutic maneuvers, such as placement of endoprostheses and passage of some dilators and retrieval baskets, require instruments with a larger (3.2 mm) channel. An adult duodenoscope with all the accessories should be available for therapeutic interventions.

## Endoscopic techniques

The duodenoscope is inserted into the second portion of the duodenum with the patient in the left lateral decubitus position or fully prone if under general anesthesia. The papilla is observed, the patient is turned prone, and a tapered Teflon catheter (3.5 F at the distal end) is introduced. An iodinated contrast agent such as 65% Uromiron® (iodamide metilglucaminic) is injected manually using a 10 or 20 ml syringe. While some endoscopists prefer non-ionic low osmolar agents (e.g. ioversol), there is no proof that these more expensive agents reduce the incidence of post-ERCP pancreatitis (5). On some occasions diluted contrast material to 30% is preferred for optimal visualization if ducts are known to be dilated or filling defects are anticipated. Meticulous fluoroscopy during injection is equally if not more important. Filling of common bile duct or pancreatic duct is monitored fluoroscopically and continuously during contrast injection.

The principles of cannulation are those used in adult patients with the additional limitations of space within the duodenum depending on age. The optimal route to the papilla is the "short route"; which involves straightening the instrument along the lesser curvature of the stomach to bring the papilla directly en face. The instrument is withdrawn slowly, keeping the controls locked and the papilla in view. This involves rotating the scope to the right while angling the tip up. In some infants it is not possible to perform this maneuver. In such cases cannulation of the papilla is performed with the "long route" in which the instrument lies along the greater curvature of the stomach. Control of the endoscope tip and elevator are more difficult in this configuration and there is more discomfort (Fig. 2.3 e and f).

In young infants, such as those undergoing investigation for neonatal cholestasis, it is important to minimize the procedure time to avoid abdominal overdistension and respiratory compromise. In our experience the mean time from introduction of the duodenoscope into the mouth to complete withdrawal is 10 minutes with a range of 2–20 minutes. To reduce the time of the procedure, the cannula is placed into the biopsy channel of the duodenoscope prior to passage, and the instrument is withdrawn as soon as the common bile duct is identified fluoroscopically. If contrast does not enter the common bile duct but only refluxes to the duodenum, or if only the pancreatic duct is visualized, the cannula is left in the curved cephalad position and the endoscope is slowly withdrawn. This may change the cannula tip orientation and straighten out the route from the papillary orifice to the common duct. Failing these attempts, lateral and vertical angulations of the cannula should be tried. It is helpful to engage the orifice with the cannula tip and then rotate the scope tip and cannula to the left, followed by cephalad orientation of the cannula tip. Deep selective cannulation of the bile duct is generally not possible for neonates given the small duct diameter.

Successful cannulation of the common bile duct or the pancreatic duct in neonates and young infants is lower than in adults. It varies from 27% to 95% according to the

*Table 1.5* Successful cannulation during ERCP in infants with neonatal cholestasis

| Author, year (Ref.) | Number of patients | Successful |
|---|---|---|
| Guelrud, 1987 (2) | 22 | 19 (86%) |
| Heyman, 1988 (6) | 11 | 3 (27%) |
| Wilkinson, 1991 (7) | 9 | 4 (45%) |
| Derkx, 1994 (8) | 20 | 18 (90%) |
| Mitchell,1994 (9) | 40 | 36 (90%) |
| Guelrud, 1996 (unpublished) | 155 | 147 (95%) |
| Total | 257 | 227 (88%) |

*Table 1.6* Successful cannulation during ERCP in children older than 1 year

| Author, year (Ref.) | Number of patients | Successful |
|---|---|---|
| Cotton, 1982 (10) | 25 | 24 (96%) |
| Kunitomo, 1988 (11) | 16 | 14 (88%) |
| Buckley, 1990 (12) | 42 | 41 (98%) |
| Putnam, 1991 (13) | 42 | 39 (93%) |
| Dite, 1992 (14) | 19 | 19 (100%) |
| Brown C, 1993 (15) | 121 | 116 (96%) |
| Brown KO, 1994 (16) | 25 | 25 (100%) |
| Lemmel, 1994 (17) | 55 | 54 (98%) |
| Portwood, 1995 (18) | 26 | 26 (100%) |
| Abu-Khalaf, 1995 (19) | 16 | 16 (100%) |
| Manegold, 1996 (20) | 38 | 36 (94%) |
| Graham, 1996 (21) | 23 | 22 (96%) |
| Guelrud, 1996 (unpublished) | 144 | 142 (98%) |
| Total | 592 | 574 (97%) |

endoscopist's experience (Table 1.5). In our experience with 155 neonates and young infants with neonatal cholestasis, the procedure was successful in 95% of the cases. The procedure was unsuccessful in eight patients because of duodenal malrotation in two and inability to cannulate in six. In older children, the percentage of cannulation of the desired duct is comparable to that achieved in adults (Table 1.6).

## Indications and contraindications

The most common indications of ERCP in pediatric patients with biliary disorders are neonatal cholestasis, obstructive jaundice, known or suspected choledocholithiasis, abnormal liver enzymes in children with inflammatory bowel diseases, abnormal biliary findings in abdominal ultrasonography and therapeutic ERCP. In children with pancreatic disorders the indications are non-resolving acute pancreatitis, idiopathic recurrent pancreatitis, chronic pancreatitis, evaluation of persistent elevation of pancreatic enzymes, evaluation of ultrasonographic abnormalities, evaluation of pancreatic pseudocysts and pancreatic ascites, evaluation of pancreatic ductal leaks form blunt abdominal trauma, and therapeutic ERCP.

Relative contraindications are severe or difficult to correct coagulation disorders. Absolute contraindications to ERCP are similar to those for upper endoscopy and include cardiovascular, respiratory or neurologic instability, and suspected bowel perforation. Severe or uncorrectable coagulation disorders are a relative contraindication, particularly if therapeutic maneuvers such as sphincterotomy are anticipated. Also, inaccessibility of the duodenum or papilla due to a luminal stricture of the esophagus or duodenum or post-operative biliary diversion, such as Roux-en-Y choledochal jejunostomy with orthotopic liver transplantation, may preclude successful ERCP.

## Complications

All endoscopic procedures carry hazards and there are risks in ERCP. The incidence of complications in pediatric patients is not well established.

Complications of ERCP in children older than one year varies according to the system studied, biliary or pancreatic. The overall incidence of complication in children is 4.7%. Buckley *et al.* (12) described 2 cases of pancreatitis in 42 children undergoing ERCP. Blustein *et al.* (24) reported 1 case of mild pancreatitis in 4 children with chronic pancreatitis following ERCP. Putnam *et al.* (13) in a series of 42 ERCP examinations in 37 children and 1 young adult, described mild pancreatitis in 3 patients (8%) all of whom had a history of pancreatitis. A fourth patient with primary sclerosing cholangitis developed fever (39°C) the night of ERCP. No patients with biliary tract pathology developed pancreatitis. Brown *et al.* (16) performed 42 ERCPs in 25 children with a variety of pancreaticobiliary indications without any major complication. Lemmel *et al.* (17) studied 54 children with recurrent pancreatitis and pancreaticobiliary pain. Endoscopic therapy was performed in 19 patients. Post ERCP pancreatitis occurred in 14% of procedures and was graded as mild in 80% of cases. One patient had endoscopic sphincterotomy-induced bleeding which was treated endoscopically. Portwood *et al.* (18) performed 36 ERCPs in 26 children with biliary and pancreatic diseases. There were 15 therapeutic interventions. One patient developed mild acute ERCP-related pancreatitis. Abu-Khalaf (19) studied 16 children with biliary tract disease without complication. Manegold *et al.* (20) had no complication in 38 children undergoing ERCP for a variety of biliary and pancreatic diseases. Sphincterotomy was performed in 6 children with pancreaticolithiasis and in 1 with benign papillary stenosis. There were 2 episodes of mild pancreatitis due to the endoscopic intervention. Graham *et al.* (21) reported 3 cases of acute ERCP-related pancreatitis in 23 children in whom ERCP was performed to study recurrent or chronic pancreatitis. Su *et al.* (26) performed 162 ERCPs in 106 children with biliopancreatic diseases. Therapeutic interventions were performed in 75 patients with 6 cases having post-procedure pancreatitis.

In our unpublished experience with 144 ERCPs in children older than one year, we had 2 ERCP-related complications (1.6%). In 75 ERCPs performed to study biliary disorders, one patient with choledochal cyst and cystolithiasis had acute cholangitis that improved with antibiotics. Of 69 ERCPs performed in children with pancreatic disorders there was one mild case of acute ERCP related pancreatitis in a patient with recurrent pancreatitis and sphincter of Oddi dysfunction. Biliary endoscopic therapy was performed in 27 patients. One (3.7%)

child developed acute mild pancreatitis and another had acute cholangitis. Pancreatic therapeutic endoscopy was performed in 31 patients. Mild post ERCP pancreatitis occurred in 4 procedures (12.9%).

## References


1. Committee on Drugs, American Academy of Pediatrics: Guidelines for monitoring and management of pediatric patients during and after sedation for diagnostic and therapeutic procedures. *Pediatrics* 1992; **89:** 1110–15.

2. Dajani A, Bisno A, Chung K, *et al.* Prevention of bacterial endocarditis. Recommendations by the American Heart Association. *JAMA* 1990; **264:** 2919–22.

3. Guelrud M, Jaen D, Torres P, *et al.* Endoscopic cholangiopancreatography in the infant: evaluation of a new prototype pediatric duodenoscope. *Gastrointest Endosc* 1987; **33:** 4–8.

4. Mauer K, Waye JD. A new pediatric duodenoscope: successful cannulation without a cannula elevator. *Gastrointest Endosc* 1989; **35:** 437–9.

5. ASGE Technology Assessment Status Evaluation: Radiographic contrast media used in ERCP, May 1995.

6. Heyman MB, Shapiro HA, Thaler MM. Endoscopic retrograde cholangiography in the diagnosis of biliary malformations in infants. *Gastrointest Endosc* 1988; **34:** 449–53.

7. Wilkinson ML, Mieli-Vergani G, Ball C, *et al.* Endoscopic retrograde cholangiopancreatography in infantile cholestasis. *Arch Dis Child* 1991; **66:** 121–3.

8. Derkx HHF, Huibregtse K, Taminiau JJA. The role of endoscopic retrograde cholangiopancreatography in cholestatic infants. *Endoscopy* 1994; **26:** 724–8.

9. Mitchell SA, Wilkinson ML. The role of ERCP in the diagnosis of neonatal conjugated hyperbilirubinemia. *Gastrointest Endosc* 1994; **40:** A55.

10. Cotton P, Lange N. Endoscopic retrograde cholangiopancreatography in children *Arch Dis Child* 1982; **57:** 131–6.

11. Kunitomo K, Ming L, Urakami Y, *et al.* Endoscopic retrograde cholangiopancreatography in pediatric biliary disease. *Tokushima J Exp Med* 1988; **35:** 57–62.

12. Buckley A, Connon JJ. The role of ERCP in children and adolescents. *Gastrointest Endosc* 1990; **36:** 369–72.

13. Putnam PE, Kocoshis SA, Orenstein SR, Schade RR. Pediatric endoscopic retrograde cholangiopancreatography. *Am J Gastroenterol* 1991; **86:** 824–30.

14. Dite P, Vacek E, Stefan H, *et al.* Endoscopic retrograde cholangiopancreatography in childhood. *Hepatogastroenterology* 1992; **39:** 291–3.

15. Brown C, Werlin S, Geenen J, *et al.* The diagnostic and therapeutic role of endoscopic retrograde cholangiopancreatography in children. *J Pediatr Gastroenterol Nutr* 1993; **17:** 19–23.

16. Brown KO, Goldschmiedt M. Endoscopic therapy of biliary and pancreatic disorders in children. *Endoscopy* 1994; **26:** 719–23.

17. Lemmel T, Hawes R, Sherman S, *et al.* Endoscopic evaluation and therapy of recurrent pancreatitis and pancreaticobiliary pain in the pediatric population. *Gastrointest Endosc* 1994; **40:** A54.

18. Portwood G, Marriatis A, Jowell PS, *et al.* Diagnostic and therapeutic ERCP in children: Safe with a high success rate in experienced hand. *Gastrointest Endosc* 1995; **41:** A342.

19. Abu-Khalaf A. The role of endoscopic retrograde cholangiography in small children and adolescents. *Surg Laparosc Endosc* 1995; **5:** 296–300.

20. Manegold BC, Gottstein T, Pescatore P. Diagnostic and therapeutic ERCP in children under 14 years. *Gastrointest Endosc* 1996; **43:** A328.

21. Graham KS, Ingram DJ, Steinberg SE, Narkewicz MR. Does ERCP alter management in pediatric pancreatitis? *J Pediatr Gastroenterol Nutr* 1996; **23:** A367.

22. Bilbao MK, Dotter CT, Lee TG, Katon RM. Complications of endoscopic retrograde cholangiopancreatography (ERCP). *Gastroenterology* 1976; **70:** 314–20.

23. Nebel OT, Silvis SE, Rogers G, *et al.* Complications associated with endoscopic retrograde cholangiopancreatography. *Gastrointest Endosc* 1975; **22:** 34–9.

24. Blustein PK, Gaskin MB, Filler J, Chai-Sing H, Connon J. Endoscopic retrograde cholangiopancreatography in pancreatitis in children and adolescents. *Pediatrics* 1981; **68:** 387–93.

25. Guelrud M, Mujica C, Jaen D, Plaz J, Arias J. The role of ERCP in the diagnosis and treatment of idiopathic recurrent pancreatitis in children and adolescents. *Gastrointest Endosc* 1994; **40:** 428–36.

26. Su AY, Hernandez EJ, Brown K, London A, Goldschmiedt M. Therapeutic endoscopic retrograde cholangiopancreatography in children. *Gastrointest Endosc* 1996; **43:** A330.

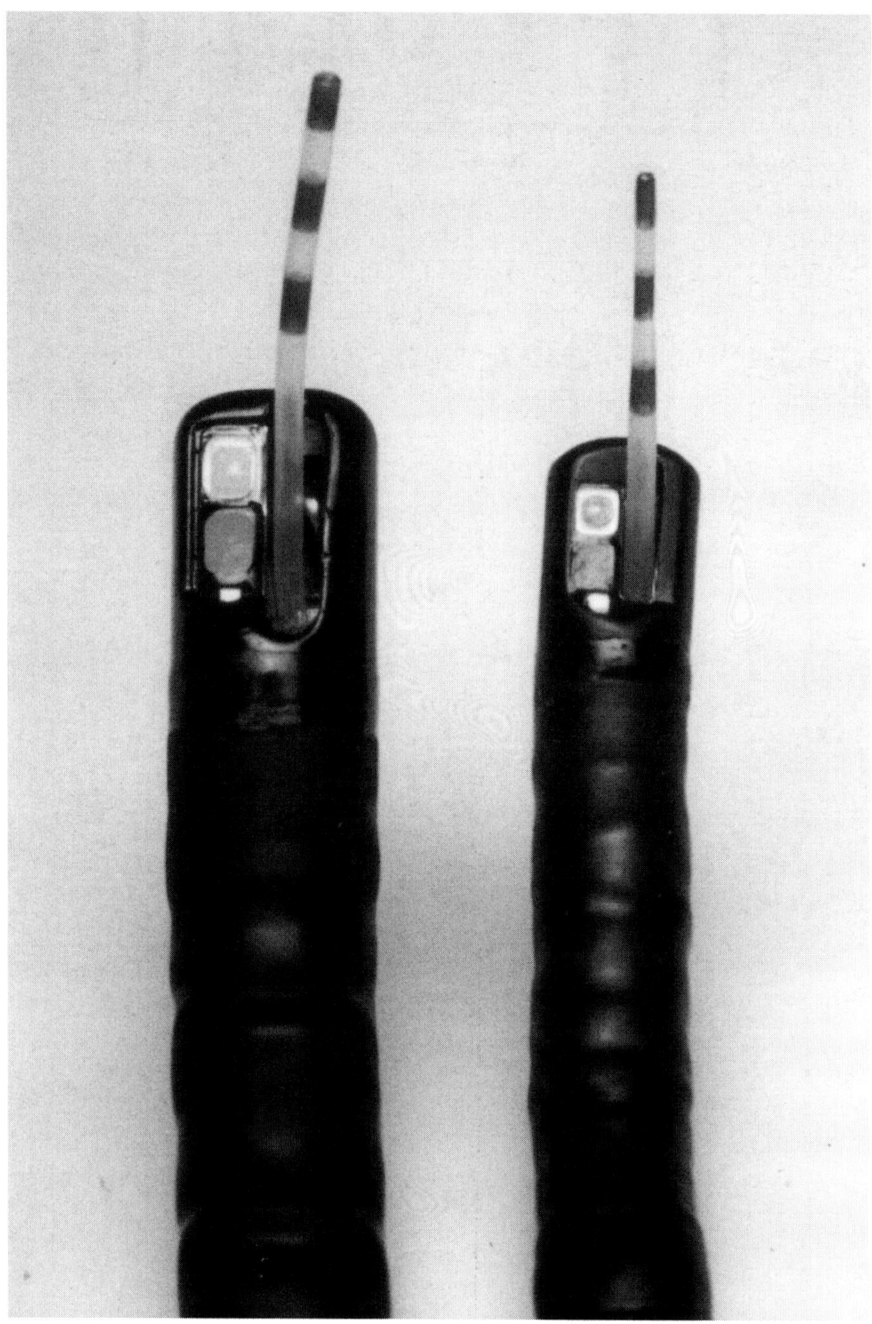

**Figure 1.1**

The Olympus PJF pediatric prototype duodenoscope with a tapered cannula (right) is compared with the Olympus JF-1T adult duodenoscope with a standard cannula (left).

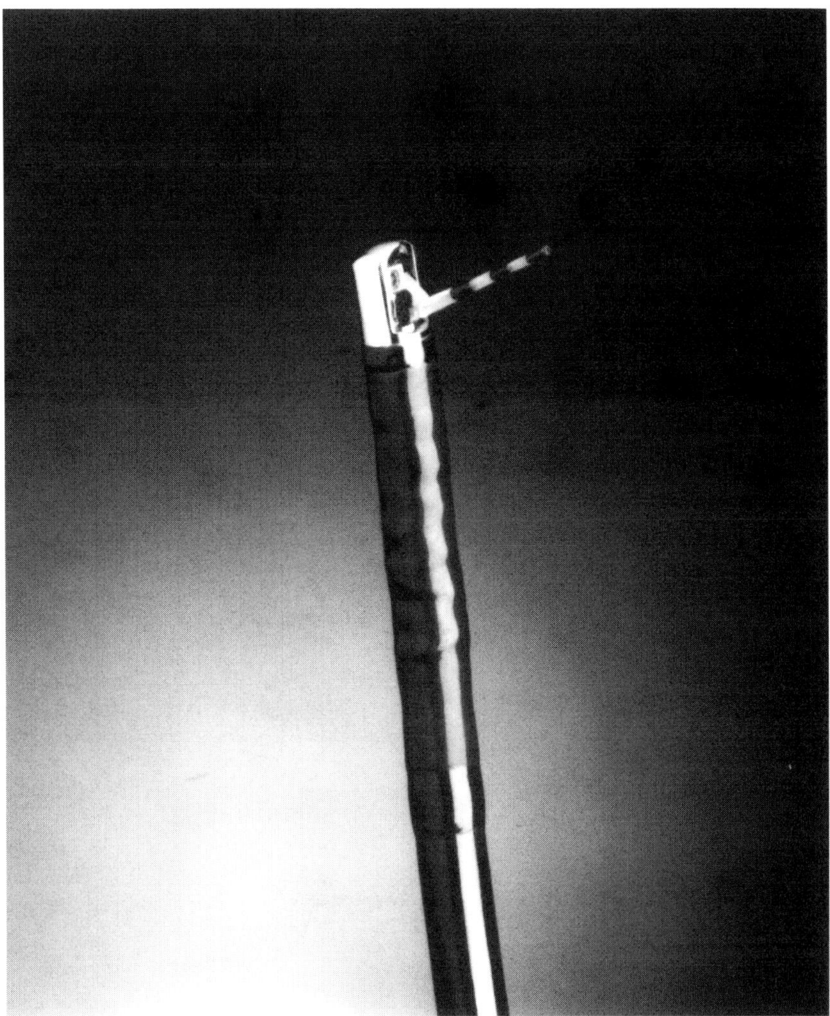

***Figure 1.2***
The newest Olympus PJF 7.5 pediatric duodenoscope with an insertion
tube diameter of 7.5 mm is commercially available.

# PART I

# ERCP in diseases of the biliary tract

# CHAPTER 2

# Congenital anomalies

## Biliary atresia and idiopathic neonatal hepatitis

Neonatal cholestasis has remained a major diagnostic challenge despite increasing knowledge regarding its pathogenesis. The causes of neonatal cholestasis anatomically range from hepatocellular injury, as in idiopathic neonatal hepatitis, to extrahepatic ductular obstruction, as in biliary atresia. Extrahepatic biliary atresia is an idiopathic, localized, complete obliteration or discontinuity of the hepatic or common bile ducts at any point from the porta hepatis to the duodenum. Jaundice may be present at birth or may appear at any time during the neonatal period. Cholestasis is diagnosed when the conjugated serum bilirubin fraction comprises more than 20% of the total (1). The clinical presentation consists of jaundice, hepatomegaly, dark urine and acholic stools that result from decreased bile flow. Clinical features and standard laboratory tests of liver function cannot reliably distinguish between diseases of the hepatocyte and those of the biliary tree. Neonates with extrahepatic biliary atresia are generally healthy full-term gestation infants with normal birth weight, although associated anomalies such as polysplenia, intestinal malrotation and congenital heart disease may be found. In contrast, infants with idiopathic neonatal hepatitis are more often products of premature delivery or low birth weight. In untreated cases, occlusion of the bile ducts results in death from hepatic failure within the first 2 years of life (2). Biliary atresia is uncommon, with a worldwide incidence reported as approximately 1 in 10,000. However, despite its low incidence, it is the most common cause of extrahepatic cholestasis in infants.

Total obstruction of bile flow leads to cholestasis, progressive fibrosis, and ultimately cirrhosis (3). The disease results from progressive destruction of the bile ducts by a necroinflammatory process of unknown etiology (4). In 1974, Landing (5) hypothesized that biliary atresia, neonatal hepatitis and choledochal cyst represent different manifestations of an inflammatory process. A perinatal infectious cholangitis leads to scarring of the biliary tract that in turn results in the sclerosis of biliary atresia. This theory is supported by the occasional association of biliary atresia with cytomegalovirus, Epstein–Barr, and reovirus type 3 infection (6). However, the role of reovirus 3 in the pathogenesis of biliary atresia remains controversial (7). Recently, it has been suggested that biliary atresia may be the result of a failure to generate an adequate cuff of mesenchymal tissue around primitive bile ducts, impairing the progress of normal differentiation into definitive adult bile ducts (8). Normally, the intrahepatic ducts originate from the ductal plate, a sheath of primitive biliary epithelium around portal vein branches which is believed to be derived from periportal hepatocytes. It has been postulated that biliary atresia results from a developmental aberration, occurring between 11 and 13 weeks' gestation, during which time the bile ducts at the porta hepatis are being formed. As bile flow increases perinatally, bile leakage from these abnormal ducts may trigger an intense inflammatory reaction with subsequent obliteration of the biliary tree (8). Despite these new and interesting theories, the etiology of the dynamic fibro-obliterative process which leads to biliary atresia remains unsolved.

The differential diagnosis of neonatal cholestasis is critical in the first 8 weeks of life because recognition of specific treatable metabolic or infectious entities will improve mortality. This will identify 70–80% of patients for whom the key differentiation is extrahepatic biliary atresia versus neonatal hepatitis (1,9). Distinction between intrahepatic and extrahepatic cholestasis is important for patient management since extrahepatic cholestasis now requires early corrective surgery with the Kasai operation or hepatoportoenterostomy for a favorable outcome. Of patients who received modified Kasai procedures by 2 months of age, 80% obtained good bile drainage (10), with 5 year survival of 54% (11). Indeed, surgery performed after 12 weeks of age may not be followed by sustained bile drainage (12–16). The Kasai operation relieves the extrahepatic obstruction avoiding rapid progression to biliary cirrhosis, but the re-establishment of bilioenteric continuity does not cure the basic disease process. Liver transplantation combined with portoenterostomy appears to be the most effective therapy for children with extrahepatic biliary atresia, and the Kasai operation offers a significant benefit by delaying transplantation (17,18).

Several procedures have been used to differentiate these entities. Laparotomy with intraoperative cholangiography has been the definitive method to establish the presence or absence of biliary atresia. The chief disadvantage of this approach is that many infants with neonatal hepatitis will have undergone unnecessary surgery to exclude biliary atresia exposing them to potentially unnecessary operative risk. In addition, exploratory laparotomy may erroneously suggest biliary atresia in some infants (19).

Duodenal drainage (20) is a simple yet highly sensitive method. If bilirubin pigment is present in duodenal fluid, biliary atresia is virtually excluded. Although some patients with neonatal hepatitis may have absence of bile-stained fluid, in the majority it will be present. Moreover, 10% of infants in whom bile is not found will not have biliary atresia. In a recent study (21), bile was observed in the duodenum in three infants with type 3 biliary atresia, demonstrating the presence of some drainage of the biliary system. Even a patient with type 2 biliary atresia has been reported having bile in the duodenum (22). False negative diagnosis of biliary atresia has been described in an infant who produced green duodenal fluid at 2 weeks of age (23) and in a 27-day-old infant previously diagnosed with neonatal hepatitis (21).

Percutaneous liver biopsy may establish the correct diagnosis of an obstructive lesion of the biliary tract in 60–90% of patients (24,25). However, the histologic features of giant cell transformation and bile ductular proliferation can be seen in both neonatal hepatitis and in the early stages of biliary atresia (26,27). In such instances, accurate distinction cannot be made. Liver histology after 2–3 months is more diagnostic although the opportunity for optimal surgical benefit may at this point be lost.

Abdominal ultrasound may be helpful (28), but the presence or absence of the gallbladder is an ambiguous finding. Non-visualization of the gallbladder may occur in association with both severe intrahepatic cholestasis and extrahepatic biliary atresia (29). Furthermore, several investigators have documented cases of patients with proven biliary atresia and normal gallbladder (30–32). Thus, although the gallbladder is usually small or absent in biliary atresia, a normal-appearing gallbladder does not exclude the diagnosis. Conversely, non-visualization of the gallbladder does not exclude the diagnosis of neonatal hepatitis or other cholestatic disorders. Guelrud *et al.* (21), found a gallbladder visualized by ultrasound in 60% of infants with neonatal hepatitis and in 25% of children with biliary atresia.

The use of scintigraphic agents has been helpful to some investigators (33–35). The accuracy of hepatobiliary scintigraphy depends on an assessment of both hepatic extraction and excretion of radiotracer. When patients are treated with phenobarbital before tracer administration, conjugation and excretion are enhanced and bile flow is increased. Biliary excretion is thus improved in patients with hepatocellular cholestasis and patent extrahepatic bile ducts. In one study, phenobarbital pretreatment identified six infants with neonatal hepatitis whose previous scans showed no liver excretion (36). Severe neonatal hepatitis can also show lack of excretion of radionuclide label, resulting in a false positive diagnosis of biliary atresia. Absent gallbladder activity is characteristic of biliary atresia on the scan, but 20% of patients with biliary atresia will have a gallbladder demonstrated on ultrasonography (36). Apparent gut excretion of radionuclide has provided false negative results of biliary atresia, which was later diagnosed on liver biopsy (37). Cox *et al.* (38) in a prospective study of 33 neonates with conjugated hyperbilirubinemia compared the results of serum liver enzymes, ultrasonography and liver biopsy with technetium-99 m disofenin scanning. When excretion of radioisotope was seen, biliary atresia was excluded, but scanning required 1 week and was less specific than ultrasonography and liver biopsy. Liver biopsy was 100% sensitive and only 87% specific for biliary atresia, and 99 mTc-disofenin scanning was 100% sensitive and only 67% specific for biliary atresia.

Ultrasonography was 78% sensitive and 75% specific. Liver enzymes lacked sensitivity and specificity for biliary atresia. The authors concluded that radionuclide liver scanning was no more reliable than the other available tests and consumed valuable time in the preoperative period.

Spivak *et al.* (35) noted in their series that only half of the patients with no excretion actually had biliary atresia. Furthermore, this proportion would have been even lower had each infant had only one scintigraphic study. Although scintigraphic proof of biliary excretion almost rules out the presence of biliary atresia, the absence of excretion is regarded as indeterminate.

The combination of several of these tests often allows an accurate diagnosis, but errors can still be made. Discriminating analysis using these variables permitted accurate diagnosis of either biliary atresia or neonatal hepatitis in 80–94% of neonates (1,16). Thus 10–20% of neonates require laparotomies to establish the diagnosis.

Visualization of a patent biliary tree in neonates, may avoid surgical explorations. In 1979 Lebwohl and Waye published the first report of ERCP in a 4-month-old infant with biliary atresia (39), using the adult duodenoscope. There were no complications and the authors felt the study would be of value in selecting infants for surgery.

The availability of a pediatric duodenoscope has facilitated investigation of neonatal cholestasis. In a series of 23 jaundiced infants ranging in age from 19 to 150 days, Ament (40) used a prototype pediatric duodenoscope (Olympus, PJF) to perform ERCP. Visualization of the biliary tree was achieved in 13 of 14 (93%) infants with neonatal hepatitis (Fig. 2.1), avoiding unnecessary surgery. In five of six (83%) infants with biliary atresia, only a pancreatogram was obtained, and biliary atresia was, therefore, suspected but not proven. In neonates and very young infants no sedation was needed. The size of these infants ranged from 2.4 to 7.3 kg. Examinations were performed quickly within a mean time of 8 minutes (range 2–18 minutes) and no complications were reported. Bile was seen in the duodenum in 12 patients, a finding felt to exclude biliary atresia, however, some infants with biliary atresia may have partial or segmental drainage.

In a larger series of 32 cholestatic infants in whom ERCP was performed with the Olympus PJF prototype duodenoscope, Guelrud *et al.* (21) distinguished three types of ERCP findings in 20 infants with biliary atresia (Fig. 2.2): type 1, in which there is no visualization of the biliary tree (Fig. 2.3); type 2, in which there is visualization of the distal common bile duct and gallbladder but not the main hepatic or intrahepatic ducts (Fig. 2.4); and type 3, which is further subdivided into two subtypes 3a and 3b. In type 3a there is opacification of the distal common bile duct, gallbladder and segment of the main hepatic duct with biliary lakes at the porta hepatis (Fig. 2.5). In type 3b, the biliary lakes are seen in both hepatic ducts (Fig. 2.6). A normal pancreatic duct was opacified in these 20 neonates. In three infants with type 3 biliary atresia, bile was seen in the duodenum. In 10 infants with suspected neonatal hepatitis in whom the liver biopsy was equivocal, opacification of the common bile duct and intrahepatic duct was obtained in all. Bile was observed in the duodenum or at the orifice of the papilla in nine (90%) of these infants and produced a false positive reading of biliary atresia in one infant with hepatic failure. The incidence of the different types of ERCP findings in 60 patients with extrahepatic biliary atresia studied by Guelrud, are shown in Table 2.1.

***Table 2.1*** ERCP findings in 60 patients with biliary atresia

| Type | No. of patients (%) | Opacification of pancreatic duct | Bile in duodenum |
| --- | --- | --- | --- |
| 1 | 19 (31.7%) | 19 (100%) | 0 |
| 2 | 30 (50.0%) | 28 (93%) | 0 |
| 3 | 11 (18.3%) | 10 (91%) | 3 (27%) |

Heyman *et al.* (41) using the Olympus PJF duodenoscope studied nine infants with biliary atresia. Three were successfully cannulated, two had type 2 ERCP findings and one had type 3 biliary atresia. Of the six who could not be cannulated, a papilla could not be located in four, one had an orifice resembling an accessory papilla which could not be cannulated, and one had a malrotation which prevented duodenal intubation. Only one of three patients who did not have extrahepatic biliary atresia was successfully cannulated.

Wilkinson *et al.* (42) used prototype pediatric duodenoscopes (Olympus PJF 7.5 and XPJF 8.0) for ERCP in nine infants with conjugated hyperbilirubinemia. They were able to prove the presence of bile ducts in four infants, obviating laparotomy. Visible bile drainage in one patient excluded atresia, and three of four infants whose bile ducts were not seen had biliary atresia.

Mitchell *et al.* (43) used prototype pediatric duodenoscopes in infants under general anesthesia. Cannulation of either the pancreatic or bile duct or both was successful in 36 of 40 patients (90%). In two of the four cannulation failures, bile was seen emerging from the papilla and biliary atresia was correctly excluded in one while the other had biliary atresia type 3 at laparotomy. In the other two patients biliary atresia was found at laparotomy. A patent biliary tree was demonstrated in 21 patients. In 15 patients the pancreatogram was normal but there was no or incomplete filling of the biliary tree so that biliary atresia was suspected. It was confirmed at laparotomy in 13 of these (87%) but in two patients no abnormality was found. Overall, in 36 patients with suspected biliary atresia, a patent biliary tree was visualized in 21 patients (58%).

Derkx *et al.* (44) performed ERCP in 20 patients with suspected biliary atresia in whom extensive investigations failed to distinguish intrahepatic from extrahepatic disease. In 18 patients the procedure was successful. In 11 patients (61%) the biliary tree was visualized and laparotomy was avoided. In seven patients only the pancreatic duct could be demonstrated. Laparotomy confirmed the diagnosis of biliary atresia in six patients. In one patient a normal extrahepatic duct was found.

In our experience during the last 12 years investigating 155 patients with neonatal cholestasis and suspected biliary atresia, the papilla was cannulated in 147 (95%). In three of the eight cannulation failures bile was seen emerging from the papilla, avoiding surgery. Each of these patients had resolution of cholestasis within 1 year. In the other five patients bile was not observed during the procedure. In four patients biliary atresia was found at laparotomy. In the other patient an operative cholangiogram demonstrated a normal biliary tree. A complete visualization of the biliary tree was obtained in 85 patients (58%), thus avoiding exploratory laparotomy. In 41 patients, an incomplete filling of an abnormal biliary tree was observed and ERCP types 2 and 3 of biliary atresia were diagnosed. In 21 patients only the pancreatic duct was opacified and atresia was suspected. This was confirmed at laparotomy in 19 (90.4%) patients. In the other two patients, a patent biliary tree was demonstrated at laparotomy.

Overall, the new pediatric duodenoscope permitted complete visualization of the biliary tree prior to exploratory laparotomy in half of the patients with neonatal cholestasis in whom the clinical, biochemical, immunologic and pathologic features were equivocal (Table 2.2), thus avoiding unnecessary laparotomies. When the biliary tree was partially visualized (types 2 and 3) the diagnosis of biliary atresia was made and confirmed by surgery. When only the pancreatic duct was opacified (type 1), the diagnosis of biliary atresia was suspected and exploratory laparotomy was indicated. Out of 147 patients, the presumed diagnosis was incorrect in only two patients (1.3%) after observations were made during attempted ERCP, i.e. including both successful cannulation and observation of bile in the duodenum.

**Table 2.2** ERCP findings in patients with neonatal cholestasis

| Author (year) | No. of patients | Visualization of the biliary tree | | Visualization of only the PD | Final diagnosis | |
|---|---|---|---|---|---|---|
| | | Complete | Partial | | Atresia | Hepatitis |
| Derkx * (94) | 18 | 5 (28%) | 6 (33%) | 7 (39%) | 6 (86%) | 1 |
| Mitchell ** (94) | 36 | 21 (58%) | 10 (28%) | 5 (14%) | 3 (60%) | 2 |
| Guelrud *** (95) | 147 | 85 (58%) | 41 (28%) | 21 (14%) | 19 (90%) | 2 |
| Total | 201 | 111 (55%) | 57 (29%) | 33 (16%) | | |

*Sensitivity 100%, Specificity 83%   **Sensit. 100%, Specif. 91%   ***Sensit. 100%, Specificity 98%

Table 2.3 shows the ultimate diagnosis in our 147 neonates and young infants with neonatal cholestasis in whom the diagnosis was equivocal. ERCP may be particularly helpful in those infants with paucity of intrahepatic ducts but a patent extrahepatic biliary tree where the results of surgical procedures, such as portoenterostomy, are poor (19).

With ERCP, absence of common bile duct opacification alone, despite several maneuvers to opacify the biliary tree, does not establish atresia. However, clinical, biochemical and liver biopsy findings in conjunction with filling of the pancreatic duct without common bile duct opacification together with absence of bile in the duodenum may be sufficient to establish the diagnosis of biliary atresia prior to surgical intervention. Clearly, the success of this technique depends upon the experience of the endoscopist, who must have confidence that non-visualization of the common bile duct is not related to technical problems and positioning the catheter. ERCP, in the hands of a skilled endoscopist, is the most direct method of establishing a diagnosis and may be appropriate as the first test when expertise and equipment are available (45).

**Table 2.3**  Ultimate diagnosis in neonates and young infants with neonatal cholestasis.

| Diagnosis | No. of Patients (%) |
| --- | --- |
| Neonatal hepatitis | 71 (48.3%) |
| Biliary atresia | 60 (40.8%) |
| Alagille syndrome and paucity syndrome | 4 (2.7%) |
| Congenital hepatic fibrosis | 1 (0.7%) |
| Caroli's disease and Caroli's syndrome | 1 (0.7%) |
| Bile-plug syndrome | 4 (2.7%) |
| Choledochal cyst | 2 (1.4%) |
| Sclerosing cholangitis | 1 (0.7%) |
| Gallstones with common duct stones | 3 (2.0%) |
| Total | 147 (100%) |

## Alagille syndrome and paucity syndrome

A variant of bile duct atresia is paucity of the interlobular bile ducts characterized by the absence of, or a reduction in, the number of bile ducts per portal triad. The extrahepatic ducts are normal or hypoplastic. This condition can occur as a part of the Alagille syndrome (46) also called arteriohepatic dysplasia or syndromic paucity of the intrahepatic ducts (SPID) in which intrahepatic cholestasis is associated with peculiar facies, incomplete iridocorneal separation, retarded growth, hypogonadism, butterfly-like vertebral arch defects and peripheral pulmonic stenosis. Differentiation of this condition from extrahepatic biliary atresia is necessary in order to avoid needless surgery. ERCP has been used to diagnose Alagille's syndrome (47,48). The cholangiogram shows marked and diffuse narrowing of the intrahepatic ducts and reduced arborization (Fig. 2.7).

We have seen three neonates with non-syndromic paucity of the bile ducts in whom the ERCP showed normal extrahepatic ducts along with irregular and narrowed intrahepatic ducts (Fig. 2.8). This diagnosis is applied to patients without the characteristic features of the Alagille syndrome whose liver biopsy indicates a decrease or absence of bile ducts. It is now apparent that non-syndromic paucity of bile ducts is a heterogeneous disorder. This syndrome has been associated with graft-versus-host disease, $\alpha$1-antitrypsin deficiency and liver allograft rejection. It has been shown that several patients with the initial diagnosis of idiopathic paucity of the intrahepatic bile ducts were later found to have typical findings of sclerosing cholangitis by percutaneous transhepatic cholangiography (49).

The prognosis of these patients seems to be worse than for patients with Alagille's syndrome (50). Because paucity of interlobular bile ducts is a feature common to many cholestasis disorders of infancy, progressive familial intrahepatic cholestasis should be considered in the differential diagnosis of non-syndromic paucity (51).

## Congenital hepatic fibrosis

Congenital hepatic fibrosis is an autosomal recessive genetic disease characterized by disordered terminal interlobular bile ducts which form multiple macroscopic and microscopic cysts within bands of fibrous tissue and preservation of normal lobular architecture (52). It is associated with autosomal recessive polycystic kidney disease (53). Hepatomegaly may be present from infancy but hepatic failure is rare. Because hepatic fibrosis has a variable clinical expression, several authors have suggested that it does not constitute a single clinical entity but rather represents a full spectrum of liver and kidney lesions (53–55). ERCP will demonstrate a normal common bile duct and irregular intrahepatic ducts with multiple small cysts in the liver (Fig. 2.9).

## Caroli's disease and Caroli's syndrome

Caroli's disease and Caroli's syndrome are autosomal-recessive genetic diseases characterized by ectasias of the larger intrahepatic bile ducts (56). In Caroli's disease, saccular dilatations are present without further histological abnormalities, whereas in Caroli's syndrome, the abnormalities of the larger ducts are associated with periportal fibrosis corresponding to congenital hepatic fibrosis (57). Both varieties may be associated with autosomal dominant polycystic kidney disease (58). The pathogenesis of Caroli's disease seems to involve total or partial arrest of remodeling of the ductal plate of the larger intrahepatic bile ducts (4).

In children with Caroli's syndrome, the clinical symptoms of cholangitis and portal hypertension may be a combination of symptoms of Caroli's disease and congenital hepatic fibrosis. Caroli's disease may be associated with choledochal cyst, the pathogenesis of which remains unknown (5,59). ERCP shows a normal common bile duct with irregular larger intrahepatic bile ducts, saccular dilatations of segmental ducts and some of their afferent branches indicating a communicating type of cystic disease (60) (Fig 2.10). The dilatation of the ducts in Caroli's disease are a predisposing factor to intrahepatic lithiasis (Fig. 2.11) which is often complicated by cholangitis.

## Cystic fibrosis

In cystic fibrosis the biliary tree may have dilatation, narrowing and/or beading of intrahepatic ducts secondary to focal or multilobular biliary cirrhosis (61) which has been attributed to intrahepatic plugging and obstruction of bile ductules. However, the recognized progression of focal cirrhosis to the more severe multilobular cirrhosis is difficult to explain on the basis of plugging of the bile ductules alone. Gaskin *et al.* (62) studied 153 patients with cystic fibrosis. Ninety-six per cent of the patients with liver disease had evidence of biliary tract obstruction, which was defined cholangiographically as a stricture of the distal common bile duct in the majority of cases (Fig. 2.12). All the patients without liver disease had normal intrahepatic and common bile duct excretion of 99 m Tc-IDA. While the frequency of these findings has not been confirmed by others, common bile duct stenosis may be a contributing factor in the progression of focal to severe multilobular disease in some patients. In such cases, endoscopic or surgical relief of common duct obstruction may prevent or ameliorate these hepatic complications. Although unproved, there may also be a role for choleretic agents such as ursodeoxycholic acid in the treatment of patients with cystic fibrosis and hepatobiliary disease (63,64).

## Choledochal cyst

Choledochal cyst is a congenital malformation of the biliary tract characterized by saccular dilatation of the biliary tree. Choledochal cyst is primarily a disease of children and young adults, and 60% of reported cases are diagnosed before the age of 10 (65). More than two-thirds of the reported cases are from Japan, and the incidence in Caucasians is estimated at less than one in 200,000 (66). The incidence is much higher among women, with a female-to-male ratio of 4:1.

Many theories have been proposed to explain the development of choledochal cysts. The more generally accepted theory proposes that cysts are acquired. The majority of patients with choledochal cysts have an anomalous pancreaticobiliary junction (67–71) and this has been suggested by Babbitt (72) as an important factor in the pathogenesis. The union of the common bile duct and the main pancreatic duct is located lateral to the duodenum up to the eighth week of gestation and then it shifts medially to lie finally within the duodenal wall. Failure of this movement could result in an anomalous pancreaticobiliary junction (73). This variant is said to be present when the length of the common channel outside the duodenal wall is greater than 6 mm (74) or when the length of the total common channel is greater than 15 mm (75,76). In several reports by different groups of investigators, 85–100% of patients had this anomalous connection (67,74,77,78). The union of the pancreatic duct and the distal common duct is located higher than normal along the common duct, outside the duodenal wall, so that it is associated with a long common channel and is therefore not under the influence of the sphincter of Oddi mechanism. According to this theory, there is reflux of pancreatic juice containing trypsin upward into the biliary system (77). Analysis of the contents of bile of infants with choledochal cyst have shown that the newborn secretes trypsin and some lipase but very little amylase (79). Therefore, reflux of trypsin into the common bile duct during fetal development can produce damage resulting in saccular dilatation of the duct (70,80,81). It has been emphasized that weakness of the choledochal wall results primarily from obstruction of the distal duct during development (82). Spitz produced cystic dilatation of the common bile duct in neonatal lamb by ligation of the distal end of the common bile duct (83). Control experiments in mature sheep produced massive dilatation of the gallbladder without dilatation of the common duct, suggesting that the weak neonatal common duct wall is responsible for the cystic dilatation. Thus, there is evidence to support the concept that distal obstruction combined with pancreaticobiliary reflux in neonates is responsible for degenerative dilatation of the extrahepatic ductal system. Todani *et al.* (77) believed that the length of the stenosis determines the form of dilatation. If a long stenosis is present, cystic dilatation is produced, and a short stenosis causes cylindrical dilatation. Studies using antenatal ultrasonography have demonstrated choledochal cysts during midgestation, which might correspond to the prolonged period of time necessary for pancreatic enzymes to damage the biliary tree (84–85). As an additional support of these theories, a positive gradient of pressure from the pancreatic duct to the cyst has been demonstrated (86). Kise *et al.* (87) reported a case of a congenital abnormality of the pancreaticobiliary union at 13 mm from the duodenum with a low entry of a dilated cystic duct into the common bile duct, presumed due to the easier reflux of pancreatic juice into the cystic duct, rather than into the common bile duct.

The normal length of the common channel in children is not known. In our experience with 58 neonates and young infants with idiopathic neonatal hepatitis the mean length of the normal common channel was 1.8 ± 0.6 mm (mean ± SD) with a range of 1.0–3.1 mm. Our maximal normal length of the common channel was 3.0 mm (mean ± 2 SD). In 32 children with ages between 1 and 12 years the mean length of the normal common channel was 3.1 ± 0.7 mm with a range of 1.8–4.3 mm. Our maximal normal length of the common channel in this group of age was 4.5 mm. Abnormally long pancreaticobiliary union has been found in 5% (3/57) of young infants with biliary atresia and in 12% (2/17) of infants with neonatal hepatitis (69). In our experience with neonates and young infants in whom ERCP was performed to evaluate neonatal cholestasis, an anomalous pancreaticobiliary union was found in 3.8% (6/156) patients. It was demonstrated in 6.8% (3/44) of patients with biliary atresia (Fig. 2.13), in 1.3% (1/76) of patients with neonatal hepatitis (Figure 2.14), and in two patients with choledochal cyst (88). The mean length of the anomalous pancreaticobiliary union was 6.9 ± 1.8 mm with a range of 4.9 mm to 9.1 mm. In 138 children with ages ranging from 1 to 19 years in whom ERCP was performed to evaluate recurrent jaundice, recurrent pancreatitis, chronic pancreatitis or pain with abdominal mass, an anomalous pancreatico-biliary union was observed in 44.9% (62/138) of patients. It was found in all of the 57 patients with choledochal cyst, in 2 patients with pancreas divisum associated with choledochal cyst and in 15.8% (3/19) of patients with recurrent pancreatitis with no other associated abnormalities. The mean length of the anomalous pancreaticobiliary union was 16.0 ± 5.6 mm with a range of 6 mm to 32 mm. There are three types of anomalous ductal union (Figure 2.15) (89). If it appears that the pancreatic duct is joining the common bile duct it is denoted as P-B type. If the common bile duct appears to join the main pancreatic duct it is denoted as B-P type, and if there is only a long common channel it is denoted as Long "Y" type (Figure 2.16).

Clinical presentation is determined by the patient's age. An infantile form of choledochal cyst is observed in children younger than 6 months. The primary mode of presentation is obstructive jaundice similar to that of biliary atresia. In our group of 147 patients with neonatal cholestasis, two patients (1.4%) had choledochal cysts. They represented 3.6% of our total of 55 children with choledochal cysts (Table 2.4). The non-infantile or adult form of clinical presentation occurs in patients older than 6 months and usually older than 2 years. It is characterized by abdominal pain with intermittent jaundice. Occasionally a palpable mass has been found. A subgroup of these patients may have recurrent pancreatitis as the primary presentation.

**Table 2.4** Clinical presentation in 55 children with choledochal cysts

|  | No. of patients |
| --- | --- |
| Infantile form |  |
| Jaundice | 2 (3.6%) |
| Adult form |  |
| Jaundice | 25 (45.5 %) |
| Pain and jaundice | 13 (23.7 %) |
| Pain, mass and jaundice | 3 (5.4 %) |
| Pain and mass | 1 (1.8 %) |
| Recurrent pancreatitis | 11 (20.0 %) |
| Total | 55 |

The anatomic classification of Todani *et al.* (90) of bile duct cyst is most often used (Fig. 2.17). The type I cyst is the most common type and accounts for 80–90% of all choledochal cysts (91). Type I is subdivided into: type A, a typical cyst dilatation of the choledochus ( Fig. 2.18); type B, segmental choledochal dilatation (Fig. 2.19); and type C, diffuse or fusiform dilatation (Fig. 2.20). Type II is a diverticulum anywhere in the extrahepatic duct. Type III, a choledochocele, involves only the intraduodenal duct (Fig. 2.21). Type IV represents multiple intrahepatic and extrahepatic cysts (Fig. 2.22), and type V (Caroli's disease), includes single or multiple intrahepatic cysts (Figs 2.10 and 2.11).

The etiology of Caroli's disease and choledochocele is not as obvious as the etiology of choledochal cyst. Caroli's disease, manifested by focal or diffuse bile duct ectasia within the liver, would not appear to have a common etiology with a choledochal cyst, but it does have an association with cystic disease of the kidney.

Although classified as one of the forms of choledochal cysts (90), choledochocele may not be related. Anomalous pancreaticobiliary union is not part of the entity. The epithelium of the bile ducts has not been described to be abnormal, and there has been no documentation of long-term predisposition towards bile duct carcinoma, which is a definite complication of choledochal cyst (92). Based on autopsy studies, Sterling (93) hypothesized that a choledochocele is an acquired evagination of the mucosa of the terminal common bile duct into the duodenum caused by an obstruction to bile outflow resulting from an impacted stone, fibrosis or papillitis. More recently, Venu *et al.* (94) and Kagiyama *et al.* (95) suggested that in some patients abnormal sphincter of Oddi motility could be a contributing factor in the pathogenesis of choledochocele. A choledochocele is a rare cause of clinical symptoms and often may be overlooked. It has been reported in association with recurrent obstructive jaundice (96) and with chronic relapsing pancreatitis (97). The diagnosis is established with certainty by cholangiography during ERCP, and because it may be small and cause little deformation of the duodenal mucosal surface, it may be easily overlooked by conventional diagnostic methods. In the past, the treatment has been surgical. However, in selected cases, a choledochocele may be effectively treated by endoscopic sphincterotomy (Fig. 2.23) (94,98).

ERCP is of significant value in outlining these cysts and their relationship to both ductal systems, providing a roadmap for the surgical approach (99,100). It is only with adequate cholangiopancreatography that an appropriate operation can be planned. Ultrasonography (101), CT, and radionuclide scans cannot provide the same quality of anatomic detail as ERCP, but these methods can provide data regarding size, contour, position and presence of stones (102). Recently, magnetic resonance has been used as a new modality for noninvasive imaging of the biliary tree (Fig. 2.24).

The presence of a distal bile duct stricture at its point of connection with the pancreatic duct is frequently observed (Fig. 2.25). It has been suggested that this stenosis leads to cystic dilation of the extrahepatic ducts (103). In neonates, because there has not been enough time for the common duct to dilate, the dilatation of the extrahepatic bile ducts tends to be cylindrical (Fig. 2.26). Primary cystolithiasis occurs in 8% of patients and usually is multiple (Fig. 2.27) involving intrahepatic and extrahepatic ducts (91,104,105). Cholangiocarcinoma (106) has been associated, presumably due to biliary stasis, reflux of pancreatic secretions and recurrent infections. An association of gallbladder carcinoma and anomalous pancreaticobiliary ductal union has also been reported (107).

The anomalous anatomic configuration of the pancreaticobiliary ductal system observed in most patients with choledochal cysts has certain technical implications in regard to management. In most patients, endoscopic sphincterotomy is probably not indicated, and endoscopic access to the biliary system for removal of stones or sludge is, therefore, not possible. In selected cases, with fusiform bile duct dilatation and widely dilated common channel, endoscopic sphincterotomy (Fig. 2.28) has been attempted with encouraging results (108). Fusiform choledochal dilatation, as opposed to cystic dilatation, has been observed to be more commonly associated with low grade, short strictures located at or distal to the pancreaticobiliary junction. (109,110). Moreover, carcinoma seldom, if ever, develops in fusiform dilatation (111).

## References


1. Balistreri WF. Neonatal cholestasis. *J Pediatr* 1985; **106:** 171–84.
2. Hays DM, Snyder WH. Lifespan in untreated biliary atresia. *Surgery* 1963; **54:** 573–5.
3. Nietgen GN, Vacanti JP, Perez-Atayde AR. Intrahepatic bile duct loss in biliary atresia despite portoenterostomy: a consequence of ongoing obstruction? *Gastroenterology* 1992; **102:** 2126–33.
4. Desmet VJ. Congenital diseases of intrahepatic bile ducts: variations on the theme "Ductal plate malformation". *Hepatology* 1992; **16:** 1069–83.

5. Landing BH. Considerations of the pathogenesis of neonatal hepatitis, biliary atresia and choledochal cyst: the concept of infantile obstructive cholangiopathy. *Progr Pediatr Surg* 1974; **6:** 113–39.

6. Morecki R, Glaser JH, Cho S, *et al.* Biliary atresia and reovirus type 3 infection. *N Engl J Med* 1982; **307:** 481–4.

7. Brown WR, Sokol RJ, Levin MR, *et al.* Lack of correlation between infection with reovirus 3 and extrahepatic biliary atresia or neonatal hepatitis. *J Pediatr* 1988; **113:** 670–6.

8. Tan CEL, Driver M, Howard ER, Moscoso GJ. Extrahepatic biliary atresia: A first-trimester event? Clues from light microscopy and immunohistochemestry. *J Pediatr Surg* 1994; **29:** 808–14.

9. Mieli-Vergani G, Howard ER, Portman B, Mowat AP. Late referral for biliary atresia-missed opportunities for effective surgery. *Lancet* 1989; **1:** 421–3.

10. Ohi R, Hanamatsu M, Mochizuki I, Chiba T, Kasai M. Progress in the treatment of biliary atresia. *World J Surg* 1985; **9:** 285–93.

11. Houwen RHJ, Zwierstra RP, Severijnen RS, *et al.* Prognosis of extrahepatic biliary atresia. *Arch Dis Child* 1989; **64:** 214–8.

12. Kasai M, Suzuki H, Ohashi E. Technique and results of operative management of biliary atresia. *World J Surg* 1978; **2:** 571–80.

13. Campbell DP. Hepatic portoenterostomy. *Am J Dis Child* 1975; **129:** 427–8.

14. Howard ER, Clement J, Driver M, Mowat AP. Extrahepatic biliary atresia. A review of 88 consecutive cases. *Proc R Soc Med* 1982; **75:** 408–13.

15. Altman RP. The portoenterostomy procedure for biliary atresia: a five year experience. *Am Surg* 1978; **188:** 351–62.

16. Ferry GD, Selby MJ, Udall J, Finegold M, Nichols B. Guide to early diagnosis of biliary obstruction in infancy. *Clin Pediatr* 1985; **24:** 305–11.

17. Stewart BA, Hall RJ, Lilly JR. Liver transplantation and the Kasai operation in biliary atresia. *J Pediatr Surg* 1988; **23:** 623–6.

18. Vacanti JP, Schamberger RC, Eraklis A, Lillehei CW. The therapy of biliary atresia combining the Kasai portoenterostomy with liver transplantation: a single center experience. *J Pediatr Surg* 1990; **25;** 149–52.

19. Markowitz J, Daum F, Kahn E, Schneider KM, So HB, Altman RP, Aiges HW, Alperstein G, Silverberg M. Arteriohepatic dysplasia. I. Pitfalls in diagnosis and management. *Hepatology* 1983; **3:** 74–6.

20. Greene HL, Helinek GL, Moran R, O'Neill J. A diagnostic approach to prolonged obstructive jaundice by 24-hour collection of duodenal fluid. *J Pediatr* 1979; **95:** 412–4.

21. Guelrud M, Jaen D, Mendoza S, Plaz J, Torres P. ERCP in the diagnosis of extrahepatic biliary atresia. *Gastrointest Endosc* 1991; **37:** 522–6.

22. Kay M, Wyllie R, Sivak MV. ERCP in the diagnosis of biliary atresia. *Gastrointest Endosc* 1992; **38:** 199.

23. Dorney SFA, Kamath KR, Middleton AW, Kan A. Diagnosis of biliary atresia. *N Engl J Med* 1983; **308:** 968.

24. Brough AJ, Bernstein J. Conjugated hyperbilirubinemia in early infancy. A re-assessment of liver biopsy. *Hum Pathol* 1974; **3:** 507–16.

25. Mowat AP, Psacharopoulos HT, Williams R. Extrahepatic biliary atresia versus neonatal hepatitis. Review of 137 prospective investigated infants. *Arch Dis Child* 1976; **51:** 763–70.

26. Ishak KG, Sharp HL. Developmental abnormalities in liver disease in childhood. In: Mc Sween RNM, Anthony TP, Schever PJ, eds. *Pathology of Liver* Edinburgh: Churchill Livingstone, 1979: 68–87.

27. Landing BH. Considerations of the pathogenesis of neonatal hepatitis biliary atresia and

choledochal cyst: the concept of infantile obstructive cholangiopathy. *Progr Pediatr Surg* 1974; **6:** 113–36.

28. Abramson SJ, Treves S, Teele RL. The infant with possible biliary atresia: evaluation by ultrasound and nuclear medicine. *Pediatr Radiol* 1982; **12:** 1–5.

29. Altman RP, Abrasion S. Potential errors in the diagnosis and surgical management of neonatal jaundice. *J Pediatr Surg* 1985; **20:** 529–34.

30. Button EM, Babcock DS, Heubi JE, *et al.* Neonatal jaundice: clinical and ultrasonographic findings. *South Med J* 1990; **83:** 294–302.

31. Kirks DR, Coleman RE, Filston HC, *et al.* An imaging approach to persistent neonatal jaundice. *Am J Roentgenol* 1984; **142:** 461–5.

32. Weinberger E, Blumhagen JD, Odell JM. Gallbladder contraction in biliary atresia. *Am J Roentgenol* 1987; **149:** 401–2.

33. Gerhold JP, Klingensmith WC. Kuni CC, Lilly JR, Silverman A, Fritzberg AR, Nixt TL. Diagnosis of biliary atresia with radionucleide hepatobiliary imaging. *Radiology* 1983; **146:** 499–504.

34. Majd M, Reba RC, Altman RP. Hepatobiliary scintigraphy with 99 m Tc PIPIDA in the evaluation of neonatal jaundice. *Pediatrics* 1981; **67:** 140–6.

35. Spivak W, Sarkar S, Winter D, *et al.* Diagnostic utility of hepatobiliary scintigraphy with 99mTc-DISIDA in neonatal cholestasis. *J Pediatr* 1987; **110:** 855–61.

36. Majd M, Reba RC, Altman RP. Effect of phenobarbital on 99 m Tc-IDA scintigraphy in the evaluation of neonatal jaundice. *Sem Nuc Med* 1981; **11:** 194–204.

37. Williamson SL, Seibert JJ, Butler HL, Golladay ES. Apparent gut excretion of Tc-99 m-DISIDA in a case of extrahepatic biliary atresia. *Pediatr Radiol* 1986; **16:** 245–7.

38. Cox KL, Stadalnik RC, McGaham JP, Sanders K, Cannon RA, Ruebner BH. Hepatobiliary scintagraphy with technetium-99 m disofenin in the evaluation of neonatal cholestasis. *J Ped Gast Nutr* 1987; **6:** 885–91.

39. Lebwohl O, Waye JD. Endoscopic retrograde cholangiopancreatography in the diagnosis of extrahepatic biliary atresia. *Am J Dis Child* 1979; **133:** 647–8.

40. Ament M. Is endoscopic cholangiopancreatography needed for the jaundice infant? *Gastrointest Endosc* 1987; **33:** 49–51.

41. Heyman MB, Shapiro HA, Thaler MM. Endoscopic retrograde cholangiography in the diagnosis of biliary malformations in infants. *Gastrointest Endosc* 1988; **34:** 449–53.

42. Wilkinson ML, Mieli-Vergani G, Ball C, Portmann B, Mowat AP. Endoscopic retrograde cholangiopancreatography in infantile cholestasis. *Arch Dis Child* 1991; **66:** 121–3.

43. Mitchell SA, Wilkinson ML. The role of ERCP in the diagnosis of neonatal conjugated hyperbilirubinemia. *Gastrointest Endosc* 1994; **40:** A55.

44. Derkx HHF, Huibregtse K, Taminiau JJA. The role of endoscopic retrograde cholangiopancreatography in cholestatic infants. *Endoscopy* 1994; **26:** 724–8.

45. Ament M. Is endoscopic cholangiopancreatography needed for the jaundice infant? *Gastrointest Endosc* 1987; **33:** 49–52.

46. Alagille D, Odievre M, Gautier M, Dommergues JP. Hepatic Ductular, hypoplasia associated with characteristic facies, vertebral malformations retarded physical, mental and sexual development and cardiac murmur. *J Pediatr* 1975; **86:** 63–71.

47. Morelli A, Pelli MA, Vedovelli A, Narducci F, Solinas A, De Benedicts FM. Endoscopic retrograde cholangiopancreatography study in Alagille's syndrome: first report. *Am J Gastroenterol* 1983; **78:** 241–4.

48. Gorelick FS, Dobbins JW, Burrell M, Riely CA. Biliary tract abnormalities in patients with arteriohepatic dysplasia. *Dig Dis Sci* 1982; **25:** 815–20.

49. Hadchouel M. Paucity of interlobular bile duct. *Semin Diagn Pathol* 1992; **9:** 24–30.

50. Alagille D, Odievre M. Gautier M, *et al.* Syndromic paucity of interlobular bile ducts (Alagille syndrome or arteriohepatic dysplasia): review of 80 cases. *J Pediatr* 1987; **110:** 195–201.

51. Alonso EM, Snorer DC, Montag A, *et al.* Histologic pathology of the liver in progressive familial intahepatic cholestasis. *J Pediatr Gastroenterol Nutrit* 1994; **18:** 128–33.

52. Alvarez F, Bernard O, Brunelle F, *et al.* Congenital hepatic fibrosis in children. *J Pediatr* 1981; **99:** 370–5.

53. Gang D, Harris J. Infantile polycystic disease of the liver and kidneys. *Clin Nephrol* 1986; **25:** 28–36.

54. Murray-Lyon IM, Ockenden BG, Williams R. Congenital hepatic fibrosis: is it a single clinical entity? *Gastroenterology* 1973; **64:** 653–6.

55. Summerfield JA, Nagafuchi Y, Sherlock S, *et al.* Hepatobiliary fibropolycystic disease: a clinical and histological review of 51 patients. *J Hepatol* 1986; **2:** 141–56.

56. Caroli J, Corcos V. La dilatation congenitale des vois biliares intrahepatiques. *Rev Medicochir Mal Foie* 1964; **39:** 1–6.

57. Mall JC, Chahremani GG, Boyer JC. Caroli's disease associated with congenital hepatic fibrosis and renal tubular ectasia. *Gastroenterology* 1974; **66:** 1029–53.

58. Jordan D, Harpaz N, Thung SN. Caroli's disease and adult polycystic kidney disease: a rarely recognized association. *Liver* 1989; **9:** 30–5.

59. Desmet VJ. Congenital diseases of intrahepatic bile ducts: variations on the theme "Ductal plate malformations". *Hepatology* 1992; **16:** 1069–83.

60. Ryckman FC, Noseworthy J. Neonatal cholestatic conditions requiring surgical reconstruction. *Semin Liver Dis* 1987; **7:** 134–54.

61. Bass S, Connon JJ, Ho CS. Biliary tree in cystic fibrosis: biliary tract abnormalities in cystic fibrosis demonstrated by endoscopic retrograde cholangiography. *Gastroenterology* 1983; **84:** 1592–6.

62. Gaskin KJ, Waters DLM, Howman-Giles R, Merl De Silva MB, Earl JW, Martin HCO, Kam AE, Brown JM, Dorney SFA. Liver disease and common-bile duct stenosis in cystic fibrosis. *N Engl J Med* 1988; **318:** 340–6.

63. Colombo C, Crosignani A, Assaisso M, *et al.* Ursodeoxycholic acid therapy in cystic fibrosis-associated liver disease: a dose response study. *Hepatology* 1992; **16:** 924–30.

64. O'Brien S, Fitzgerald MX, Hegarty JE. A controlled trial of ursodeoxycholic acid treatment in cystic fibrosis-related liver disease. *Eur J Gastroenterol Hepatol* 1992; **4:** 857–63.

65. Yamaguchi M. Congenital choledochal cyst: analysis of 1433 patients in the Japanese literature. *Am J Surg* 1980; **140:** 653–7.

66. Deeg HJ, Rominger JM, Shah AN. Choledochal cyst and pancreatic carcinoma demonstrated simultaneously by endoscopic retrograde cholangiopancreatography. *South Med J* 1980; **73:** 1678–9.

67. Guelrud M, Jaen D, Mendoza S, Torres P. Usefulness of endoscopic retrograde cholangiopancreatography in diagnosis of choledochal cysts in children. *GEN* 1989; **43:** 9–12.

68. Kimura K, Ohto M, Ono T, *et al.* Congenital cystic dilatation of the common bile duct. Relationship to anomalous pancreaticobiliary ductal union. *Am J Roentgenol* 1977; **928:** 571–7.

69. Arima E, Akita H. Congenital biliary tract dilatation and anomalous junction of the pancreaticobiliary system. *J Pediatr Surg* 1979; **14:** 9–15.

70. Oguchi Y, Okada A, Nakamura T, *et al.* Histopathologic studies of congenital dilatation of the bile duct as related to an anomalous junction of the pancreaticobiliary ductal system: clinical and experimental studies. *Surgery* 1988; **103:** 168–173.

71. Ikada A, Nakamura T, Higaki J, *et al.* Congenital dilatation of the bile duct in 100 instances and its relationship with anomalous junction. *Surg Gynecol Obstet* 1990; **171:** 291–8.

72. Babbitt DP. Congenital choledochal cysts: new etiological concept based on anomalous relationship of common bile duct and pancreatic bulb. *Ann Radiol* 1969; **12:** 231–40.

73. Wong KC, Lister J. Human fetal development of hepatopancreatic duct junction. A possible explanation of congenital dilatation of the biliary tract. *J Pediatr Surg* 1981; **16:** 139–45.

74. Ono J, Sakoda K, Akita H. Surgical aspects of cystic dilatation of the bile duct-an anomalous junction of the pancreaticobiliary tract in adults. *Ann Surg* 1982; **195:** 203–8.

75. Kimura K, Ohto M, Saisho H, Unozawa T, Tsuchiya Y, Morita M, Ebara M, Matsutani S, Okuda K. Association of gallbladder carcinoma and anomalous pancreaticobiliary ductal union. *Gastroenterology* 1985; **89:** 1258–65.

76. Misra SP, Gulati P, Thorat VK, *et al.* Pancreaticobiliary ductal union in biliary diseases. An endoscopic retrograde cholangiopancreatography study. *Gastroenterology* 1989; **96:** 907–12.

77. Todani T, Watanabe Y, Fujii T, Ukemura S. Anomalous arrangement of the pancreaticobiliary ductal system in patients with a choledochal cyst. *Am J Surg* 1984; **147:** 672–6.

78. Thatcher BS, Sivak MV, Hermann RE, Esselstyn CB. ERCP in evaluation and diagnosis of choledochal cyst: report of five cases. *Gastrointest Endosc* 1986; **32:** 27–31.

79. O'Neill JA. Choledochal cyst, in Welch KJ, Randolph JG, Ravitch MM, *et al.* (eds): *Pediatr Surgery.* Chicago, Year Book Medical Publishing, 1987: 1056–60.

80. Yamashiro Y. Experimental study of the pathogenesis of choledochal cyst and pancreatitis with special reference to the role of bile acids and pancreatic enzymes in the anomalous choledochopancreatico ductal junction. *J Pediatr Gastroenterol Nutr* 1984; **3:** 721–7.

81. Narita H, Hashimoto T, Suzuki T, *et al.* Clinical and experimental studies on the activation mechanism of pancreatic enzyme refluxing into the biliary tract with an anomalous pancreaticobiliary ductal junction. *J Jpn Soc Pediatr Surg* 1990; **26:** 609–15.

82. Miyano T, Suruga K, Chen SC. A clinicopathologic study of choledochal cyst. *World J Surg* 1980; **4:** 431–8.

83. Spitz L. Experimental production of cystic dilatation of the common bile duct in neonatal lambs. *J Pediatr Surg* 1977; **12:** 39–42.

84. Dewbury KC, Aluwuhare ARP, Burch SJ, *et al.* Prenatal ultrasound demonstration of a choledochal cyst. *Br J Radiol* 1980; **53:** 906–7.

85. Bancroft JD, Bucuvalas JC, Ryckman FC, *et al.* Antenatal diagnosis of choledochal cyst. *J Pediatr Gastroenterol Nutr* 1994; **18:** 142–5.

86. Tanaka M, Ikeda S, Kawakami K, Nakayama F. The presence of positive pressure gradient from pancreatic duct to choledochal cyst demonstrated by duodenoscopic microtransducer manometry: clue to pancreaticobiliary reflux. *Endoscopy* 1982; **14:** 45–7.

87. Kise Y, Uetsuji S, Takada H, Yamamura M, Yamamoto M. Dilatation of the cystic duct with its congenital low entry into the common hepatic duct. *Am J Gastroenterol* 1990; **85:** 769–70.

88. Guelrud M, Morera C, Rodriguez M, Prados JG, Jaen D. ERCP in the evaluation and diagnosis of anomalous pancreaticobiliary junction in childhood. *Gastrointest Endosc* 1996; **43:** A327.

89. Misra SP, Dwivedi M. Pancreaticobiliary ductal union. *Gut* 1990; **31:** 1144–9.

90. Todani T, Watanabe Y, Narusue M. Congenital bile duct cyst. *Am J Surg* 1977; **134:** 263–9.

91. Yamaguchi M. Congenital choledochal cyst: analysis of 1433 patients in the Japanese literature. *Am J Surg* 1980; **140:** 653–7.

92. Gupta S, Kumar A, Gupta S, Carcinoma in choledochal cyst. *J Surg Oncol* 1981; **16:** 313–8.

93. Sterling JA. Diverticula in the terminal portion of the common bile duct. *Am J Pathol* 1949; **25:** 325–35.

94. Venu RP, Geenen JE, Hogan WJ, Dodds WJ, Wilson SW, Stewart ET, Soergel KH. Role of endoscopic retrograde cholangiopancreatography in the diagnosis and treatment of choledochocele. *Gastroenterology* 1984; **87:** 1144–9.

95. Kagiyama S, Okazaki K, Yamamoto Y, Yamamoto Y. Anatomic variants of choledochocele and manometric measurements of pressure in the cele and the orifice zone. *Am J Gastroenterol* 1987; **82:** 641–9.

96. Marshall JB, Halpin TC. Choledochocele as the cause of recurrent obstructive jaundice in childhood: diagnosis by ERCP. *Gastrointest Endosc* 1982; **28:** 88–90.

97. Greene FL, Brown JJ, Rubinstein P, Anderson MC. Choledochocele and recurrent pancreatitis. Diagnosis and surgical management. *Am J Surg* 1985; **149:** 306–9.

98. Siegel JH, Harding GT, Chateau F. Endoscopic incision of choledochal cyst (choledochocele). *Endoscopy* 1981; **13:** 200–2.

99. Jona JZ, Babbit DP, Starshak RJ, LaPorta AJ, Glicklich M, Cohen RD. Anatomic observations and etiologic and surgical considerations in choledochal cysts. *J Pediatr Surg* 1979; **14:** 315–20.

100. Anand AC, Sahni P, Dip NB, Vashisht S, Tandon RK. Congenital biliary cysts in Indian adults. *Am J Gastroenterol* 1991; **86:** 850–3.

101. Little KH, Loeb PM. Choledochal cyst. *S Med J* 1989; **82:** 255–8.

102. Chang M, Wang T, Chen C, Hung W. Congenital bile duct dilatation in children. *J Pediatr Surg* 1986; **21:** 112–7.

103. O'Neill JA, Jr. Choledochal cyst. In: Wells SA, Jr, ed. *Current Problems in Surgery.* St. Louis: Mosby Year Book, Inc., 1992: 363–410.

104. Sherman P, Kolster E, Davies C, Stringer D, Weber J. Choledochal cysts: heterogeneity of clinical presentation. *J Pediatr Gastroenterol Nutr* 1986; **5:** 867–72.

105. Lilly JR. The surgical treatment of choledochal cysts. *Surg Gynecol Obstet* 1979; **149:** 36–42.

106. Bloustein PA. Association of carcinoma with congenital cystic conditions of the liver and bile ducts. *Am J Gastroenterol* 1977; **67:** 40–6.

107. Kimura K, Ohto M, Saisho H, Unozawa T, Tsuchiya Y, Morita M, Ebara M, Matsutani S, Okuda K. Association of gallbladder carcinoma and anomalous pancreaticobiliary ductal union. *Gastroenterology* 1985; **89:** 1258–65.

108. NG WD, Liu K, Wong MK, *et al.* Endoscopic sphincterotomy in young patients with choledochal dilatation and a long common channel: a preliminary report. *Br J Surg* 1992; **79:** 550–2.

109. Todani T, Watanabe Y, Fujii T, *et al.* Anomalous arrangement of the pancreaticobiliary ductal system in patients with a choledochal cyst. Am J Surg 1984; **147:** 672–7.

110. Ito T, Ando M, Nagaya T, Sugito T. Congenital dilatation of the common bile duct in children. The etiologic significance of the narrow segment distal to the dilated common bile duct. *Z Kinderchir* 1984; **30:** 40–5.

111. Todani T, Watanabe Y, Fujii, *et al.* Cylindrical dilatation of the choledochus: a special type of congenital bile duct dilatation. *Surgery* 1985; **98:** 964–8.

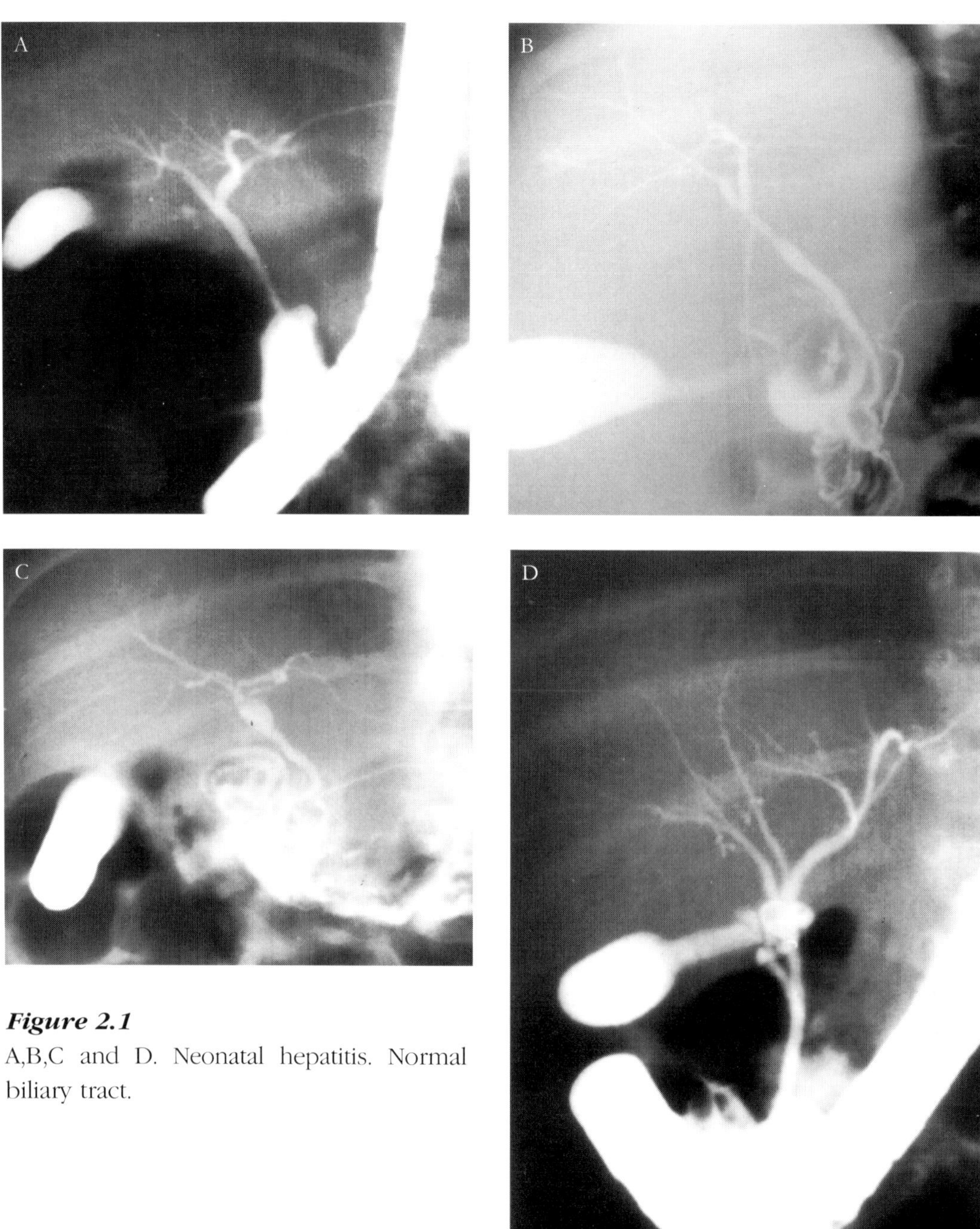

***Figure 2.1***
A,B,C and D. Neonatal hepatitis. Normal biliary tract.

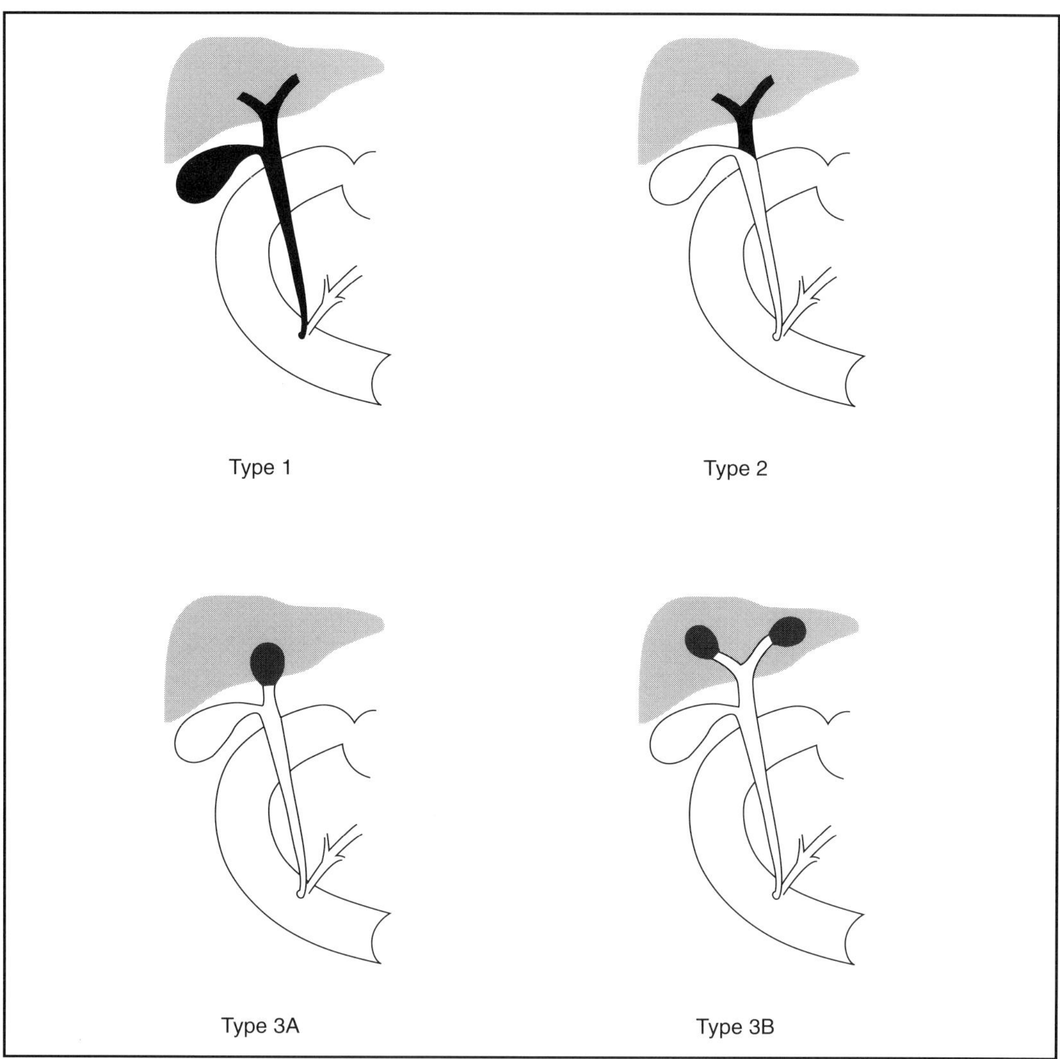


**Figure 2.2**

Schematic representation of ERCP radiological findings in biliary atresia. Type 1: no visualization of biliary tree. Type 2: opacification of the distal common duct and gallbladder without visualization of the main hepatic duct. Type 3 is divided in two subtypes. Type 3A: opacification of the distal common duct, gallbladder and segment of the main hepatic duct with biliary lakes at the porta hepatis. Type 3B: the biliary lakes are seen in both hepatic ducts.

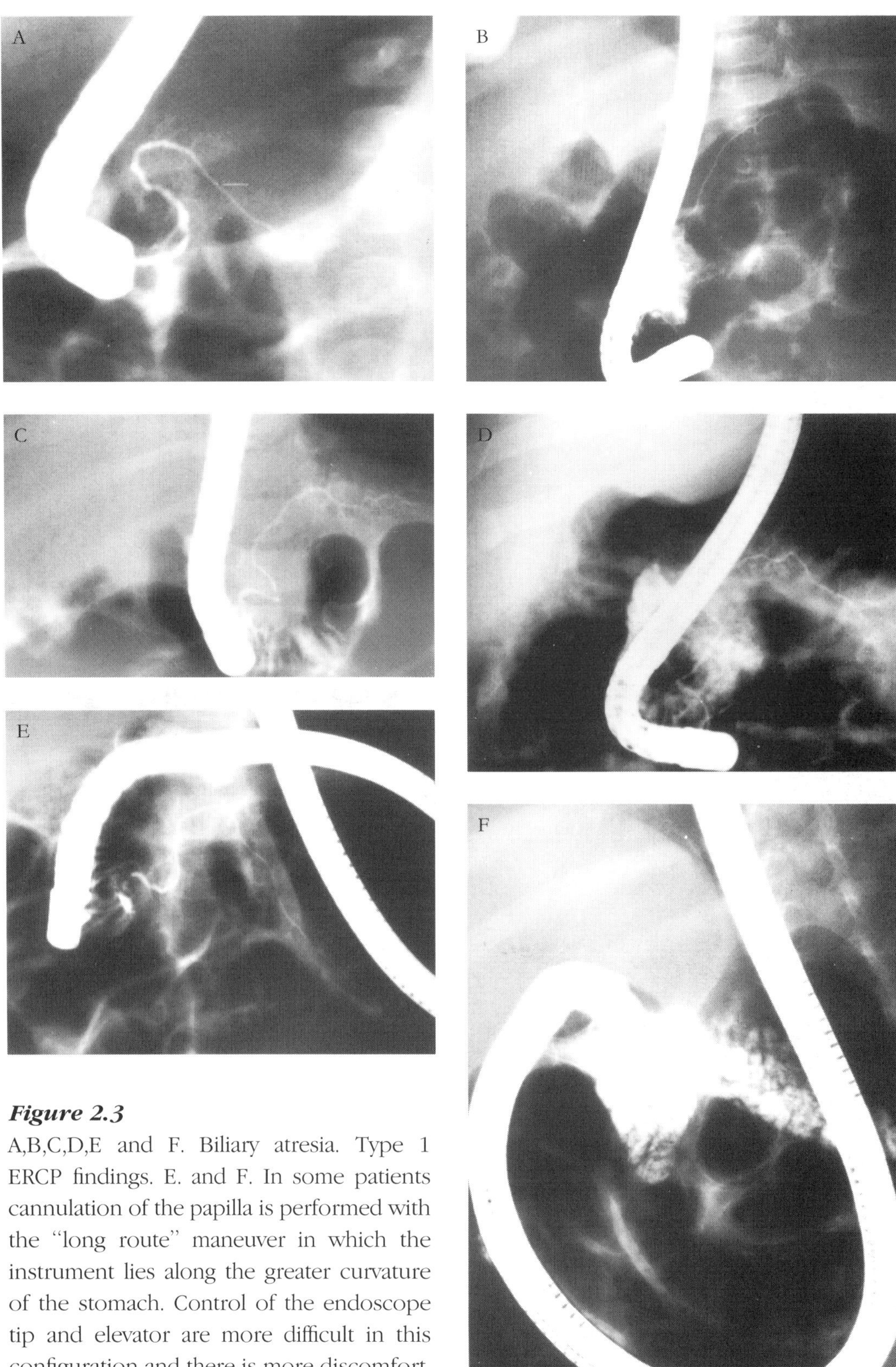

***Figure 2.3***
A,B,C,D,E and F. Biliary atresia. Type 1
ERCP findings. E. and F. In some patients
cannulation of the papilla is performed with
the "long route" maneuver in which the
instrument lies along the greater curvature
of the stomach. Control of the endoscope
tip and elevator are more difficult in this
configuration and there is more discomfort.

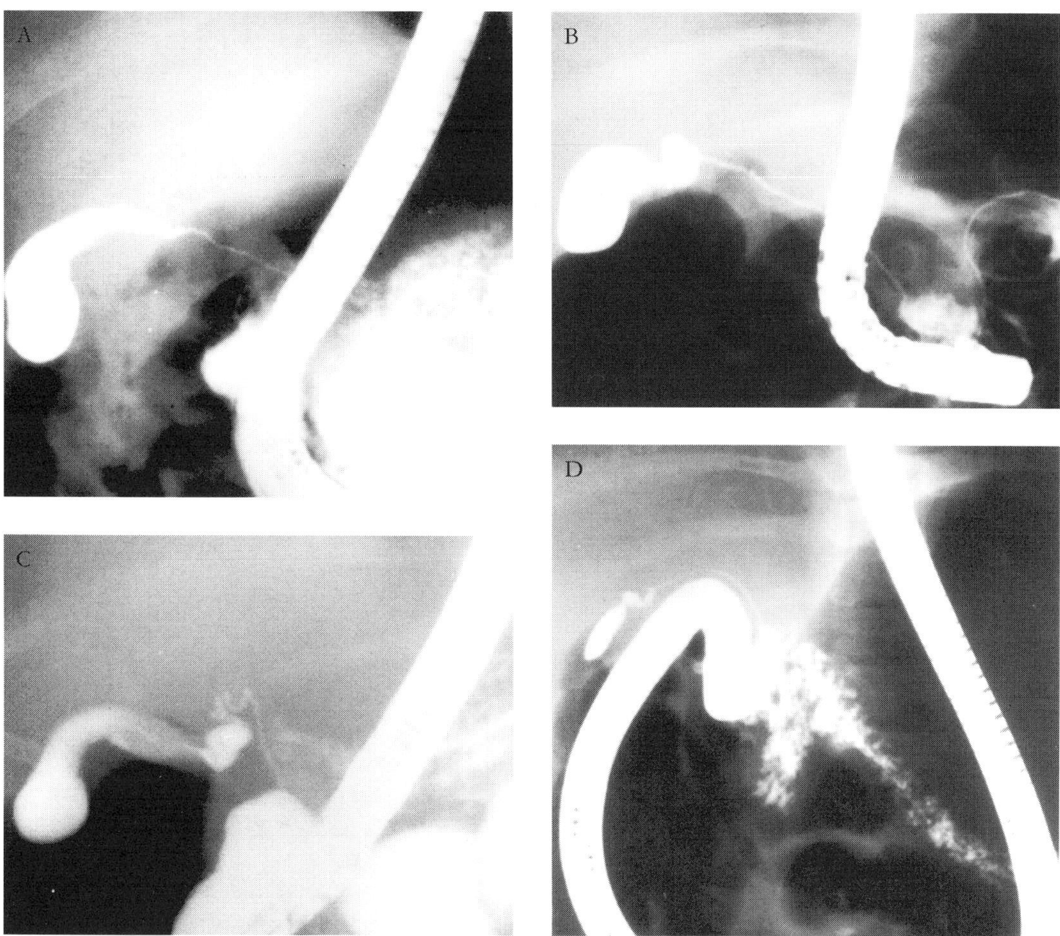

**_Figure 2.4_**
A,B,C and D. Biliary atresia. Type 2 ERCP findings.

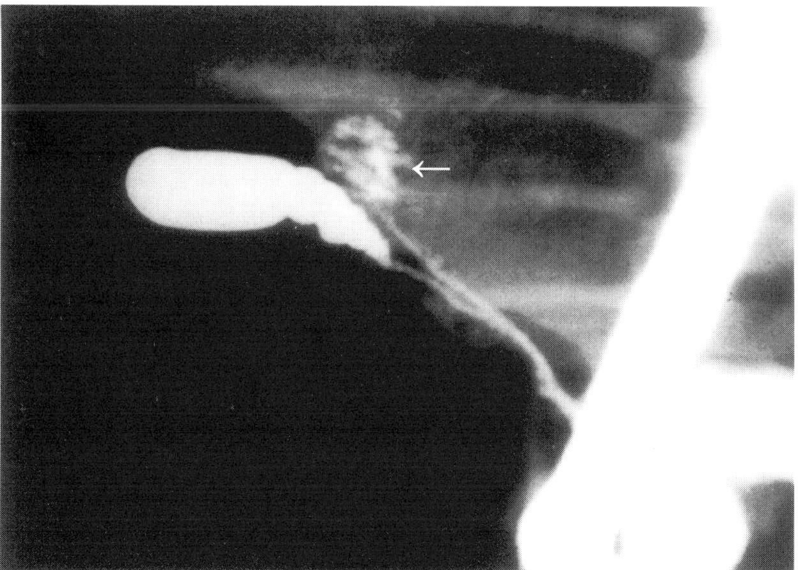

**_Figure 2.5_** Biliary atresia. Type 3A ERCP findings. 25-day-old neonate. Distal, irregular, narrowed common bile duct and common hepatic duct. Multiple "biliary lakes" at the porta hepatis (↑). Normal gallbladder.

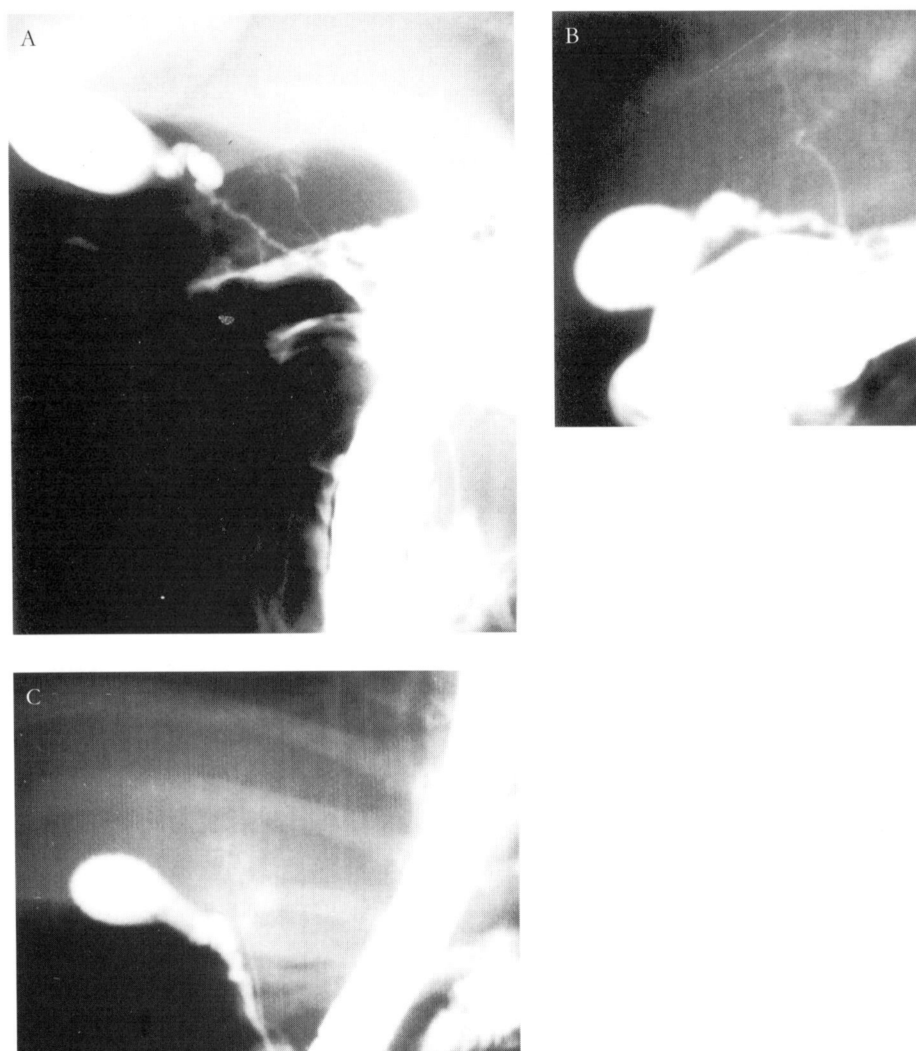

***Figure 2.6***
A,B and C. Biliary atresia. Type 3B ERCP findings.

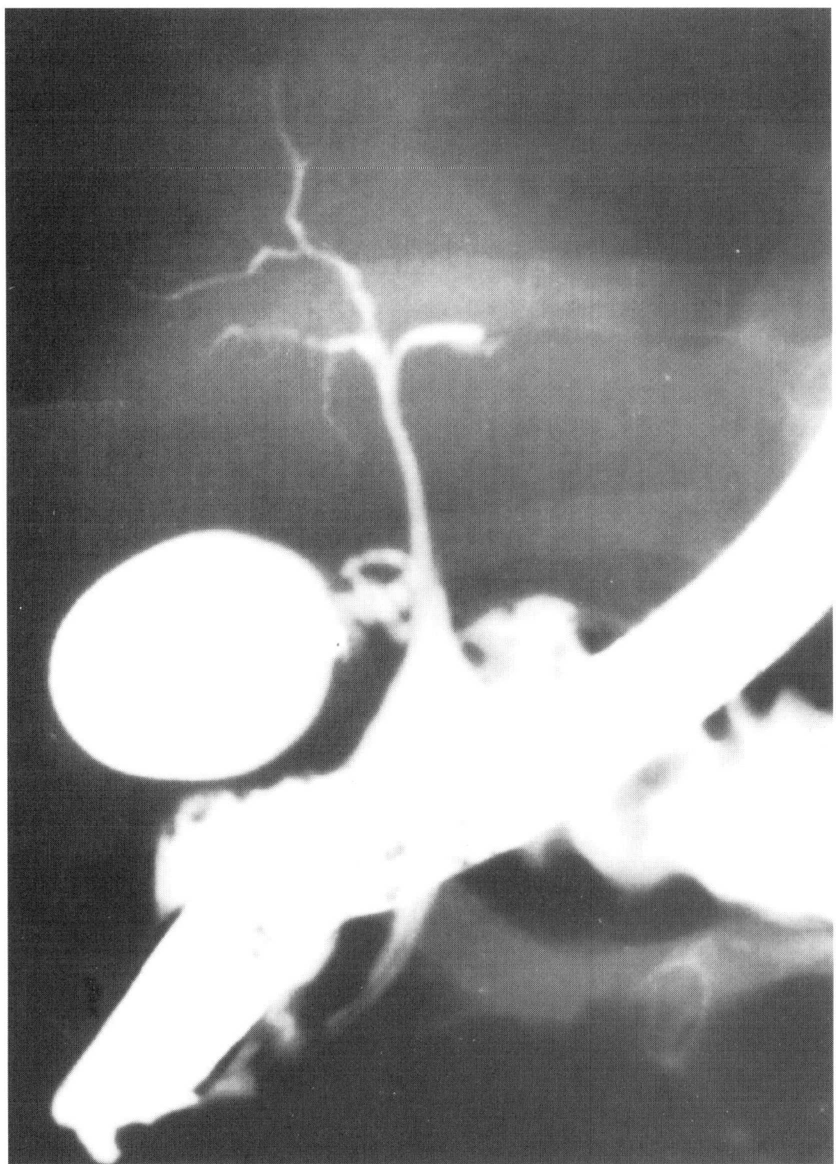

***Figure 2.7***
Alagille syndrome in a 2-year-old female infant with peripheral pulmonary artery stenosis and butterfly-like vertebral arch defects. Normal extrahepatic ducts. Diminished and narrowed intrahepatic ducts.

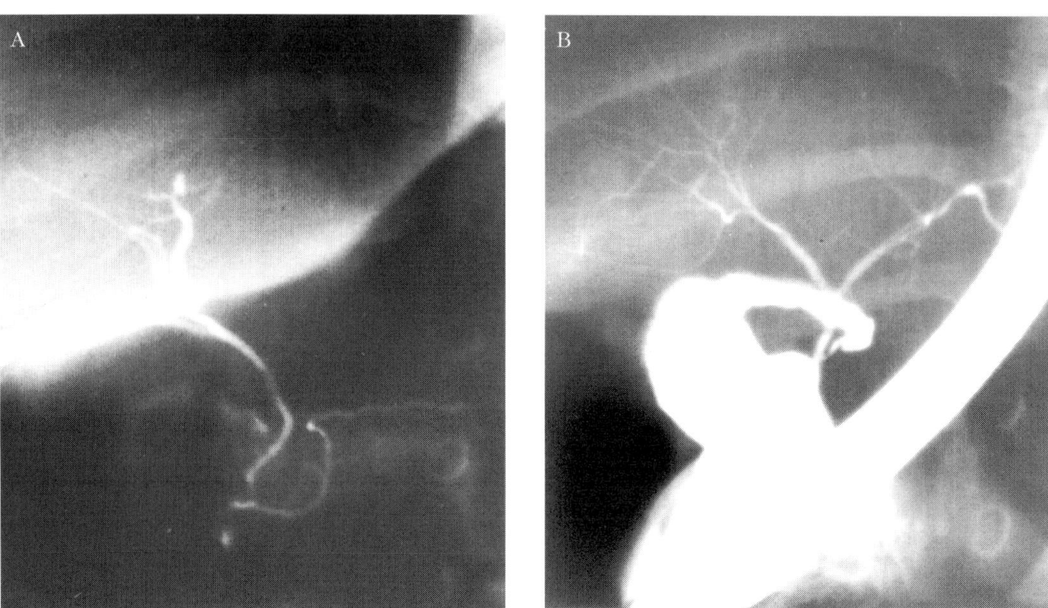

**Figure 2.8**
(A) Non-syndromatic paucity of bile ducts in a 4-month-old male infant. Normal extrahepatic ducts. Narrowed intrahepatic ducts. (B) Non-syndromatic paucity of bile ducts in a 62-day-old young infant. Normal extrahepatic ducts. Narrowed intrahepatic ducts.

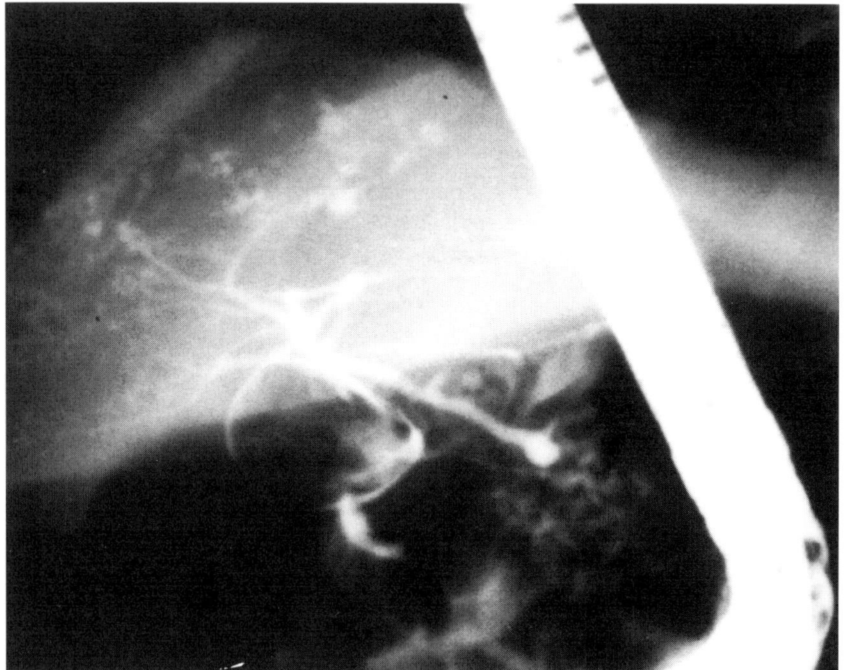

**Figure 2.9**
Congenital hepatic fibrosis in a 38-day-old young infant with cholestasis. Normal extrahepatic ducts. Irregular and narrowed intrahepatic ducts. Multiple small cysts in the liver.

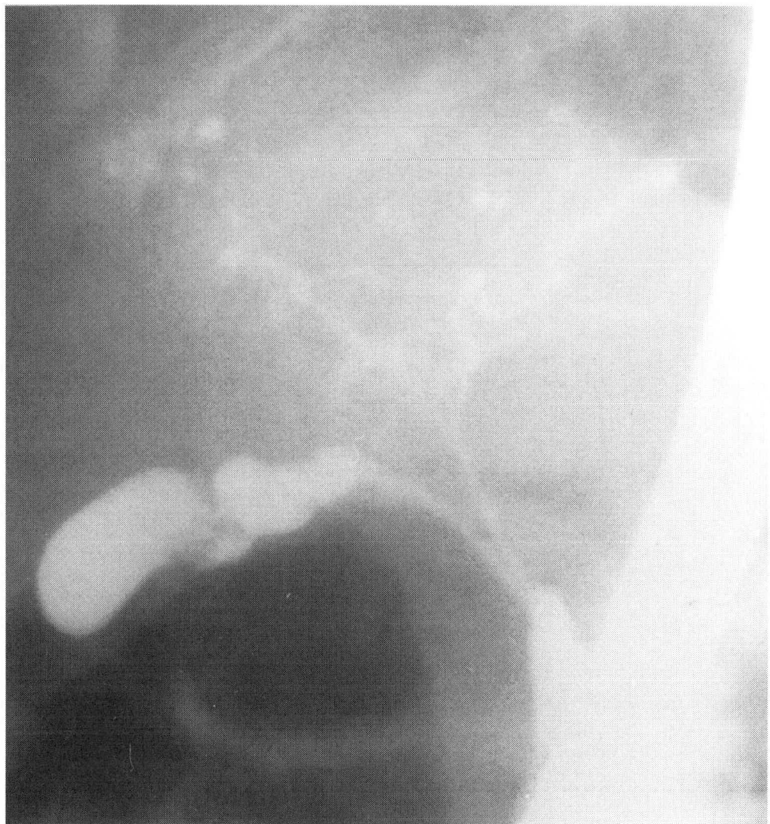

**Figure 2.10**
Caroli's syndrome with hepatic fibrosis in a 21-month-old infant.
Normal extrahepatic ducts. Segmental cystic-like dilatation of larger
intrahepatic ducts.

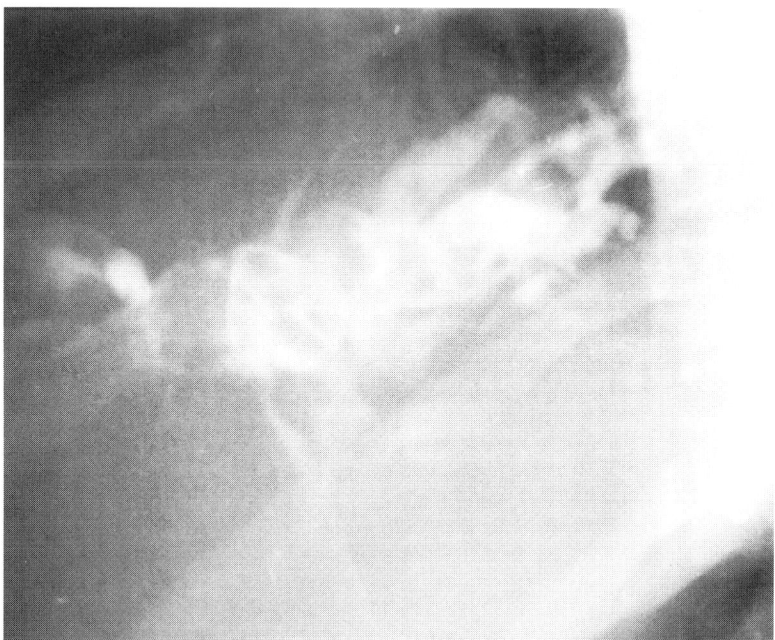

**Figure 2.11**
Caroli's disease with intraductal lithiasis in a 6-year-old male.
Normal extrahepatic ducts. Irregular larger intrahepatic bile ducts
with saccular dilatation of segmental ducts and of their afferent
branches. Multiple intraductal lithiasis.

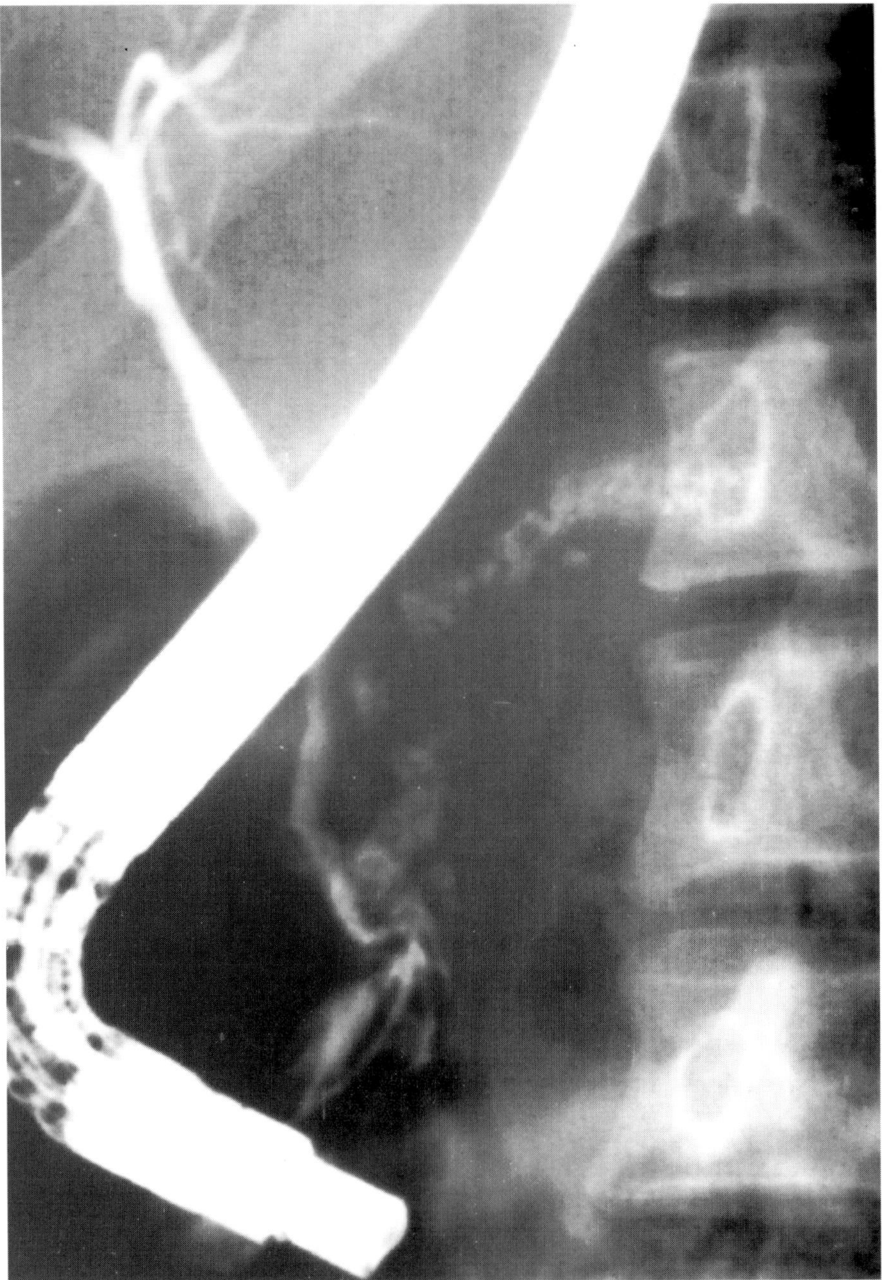

***Figure 2.12***
Cystic fibrosis and chronic pancreatitis in a 9-year-old female. Irregular common bile duct in its intrapancreatic segment due to encasement of chronic pancreatitis. Multiple pancreatic calcifications.

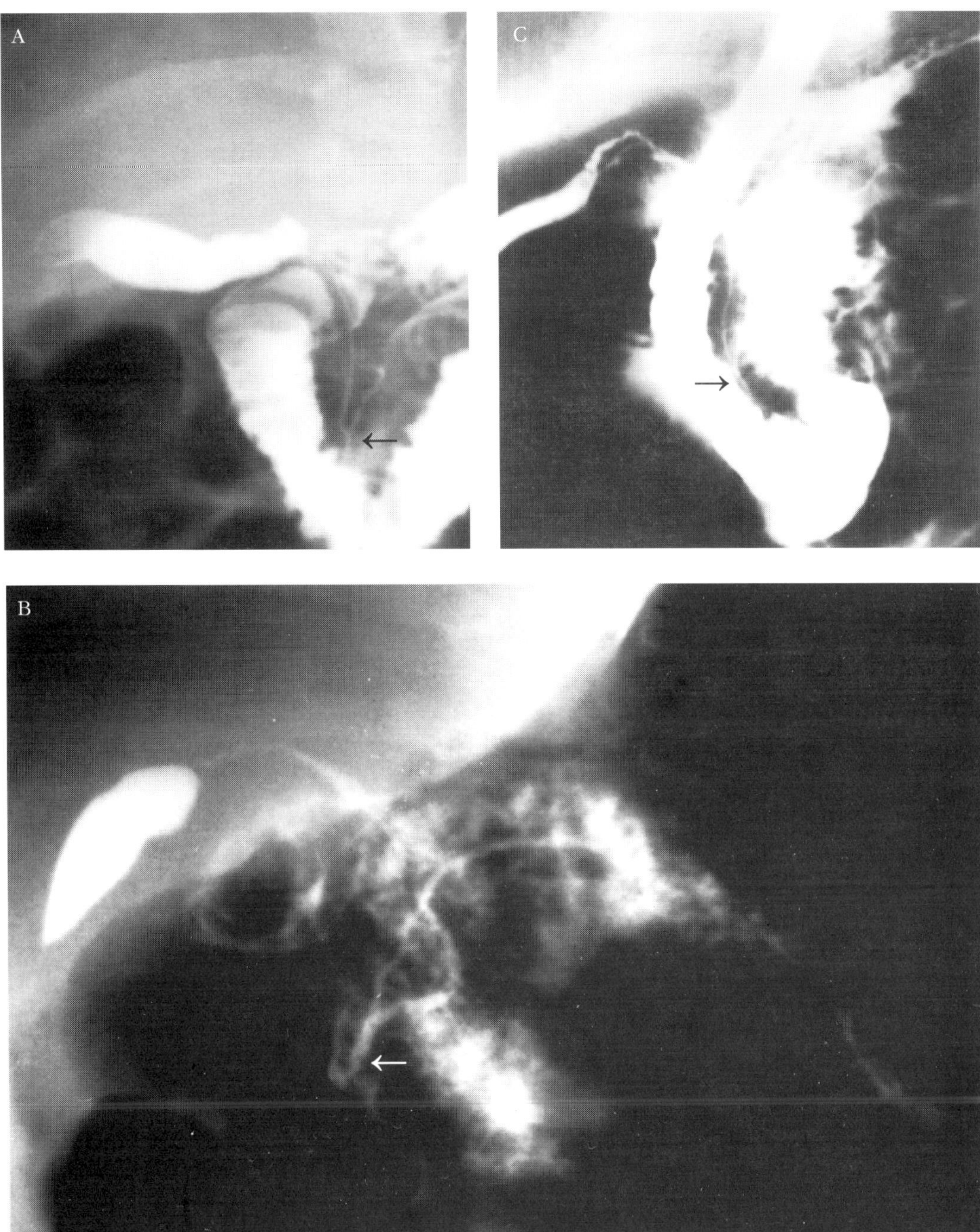

***Figure 2.13***

Anomalous pancreaticobiliary union (APBU) and biliary atresia. (A) Type 2 ERCP findings in a 30-day-old female neonate. Normal distal common duct and gallbladder. Long APBU (↑). (B) Type 2 ERCP findings in a 43-day-old young female infant. Long APBU (↑). The pancreatic duct is slightly dilated when compared with the common duct. Normal gallbladder without hepatic ducts visualization. (C) Type 2 ERCP findings in a 36-day-old young infant. Normal pancreatic duct. Narrowed and irregular distal common duct with normal gallbladder. Long APBU (↑).

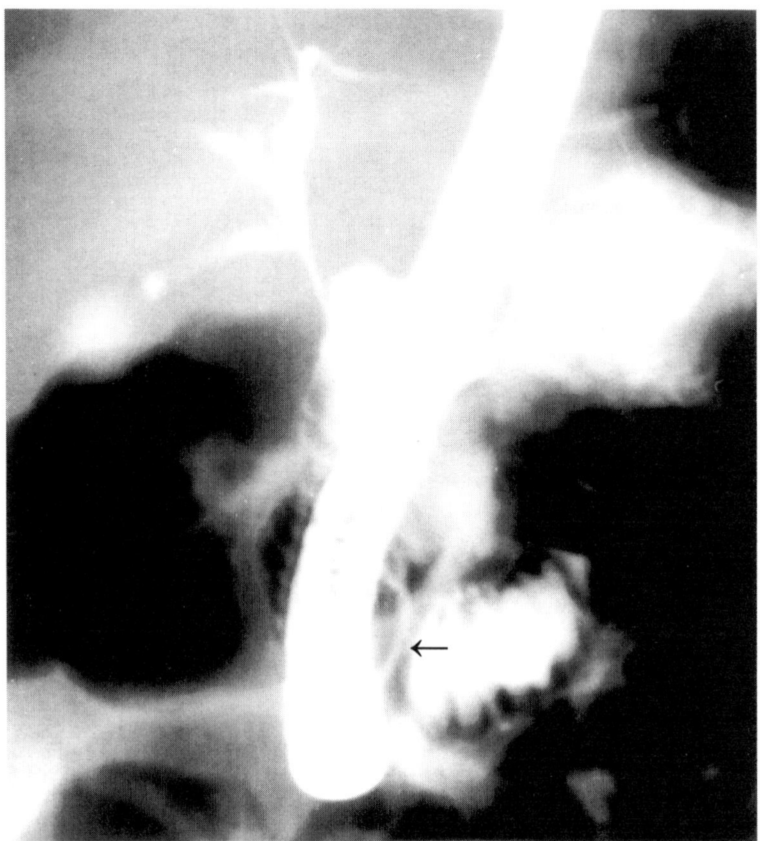

**Figure 2.14**

Anomalous pancreaticobiliary union and neonatal hepatitis in a 40-day-old young infant. Normal pancreatic duct. Slightly dilated right and left extrahepatic ducts. Long APBU (↑).

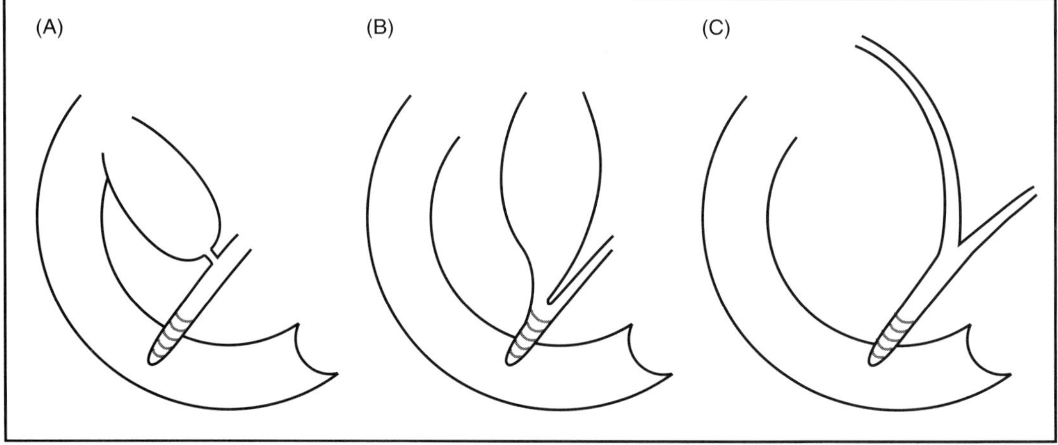

**Figure 2.15**

Schematic representation of anomalous pancreaticobiliary union. (A) BP type: the common bile duct appears to join the pancreatic duct. (B) PB type: the pancreatic duct appears to join the common bile duct. (C) Long "Y" type: there is only a long common channel.

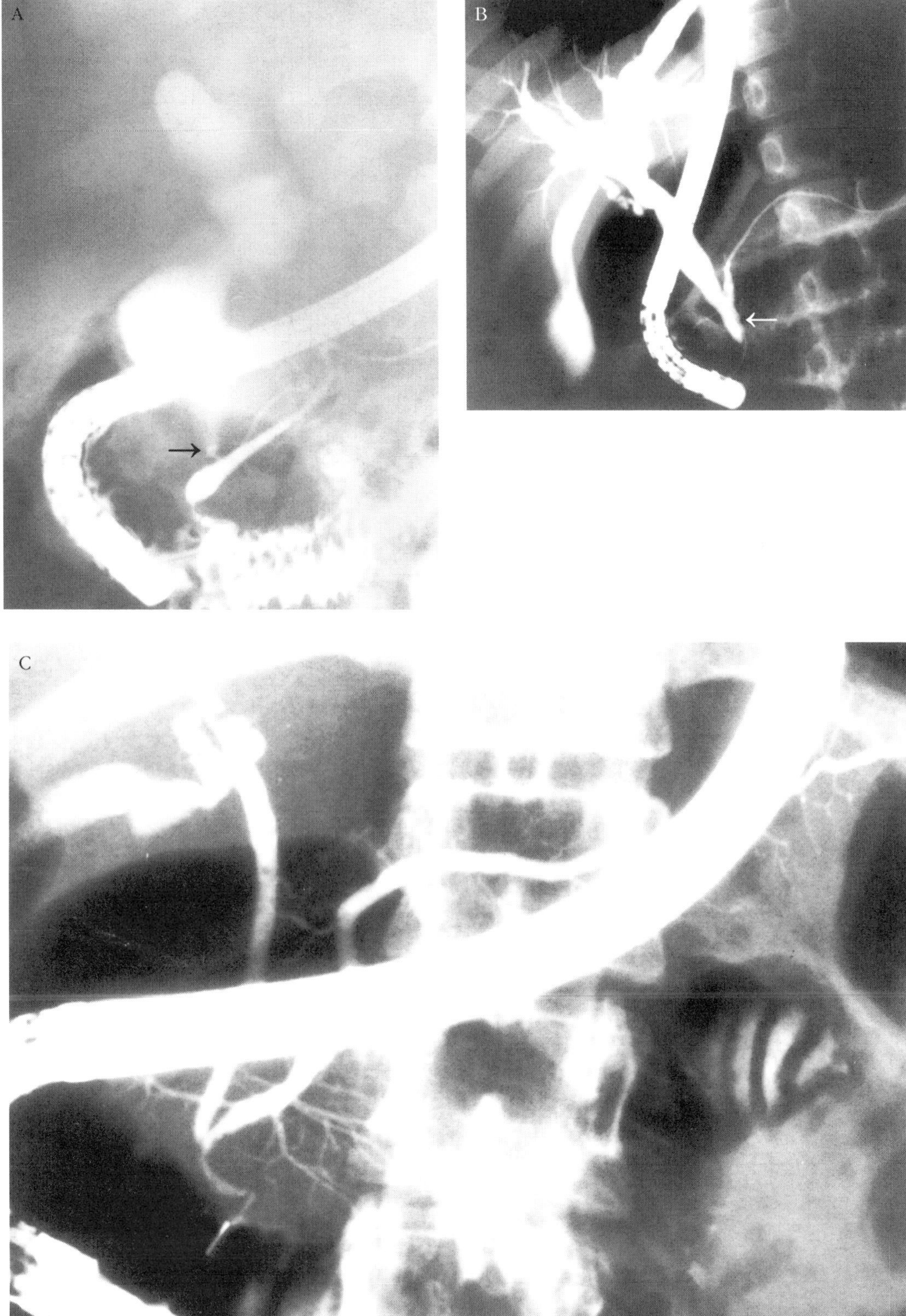

***Figure 2.16***

Anomalous pancreaticobiliary union. (A) Type BP union in a 12-year-old female with a choledochal cyst type IV A (↑). Note a stricture at the most distal segment of the common duct. (B) Type PB union (↑) in a 4-year-old female with type IV A choledochal cyst. (C) Long "Y" type union in a 15-year-old female.

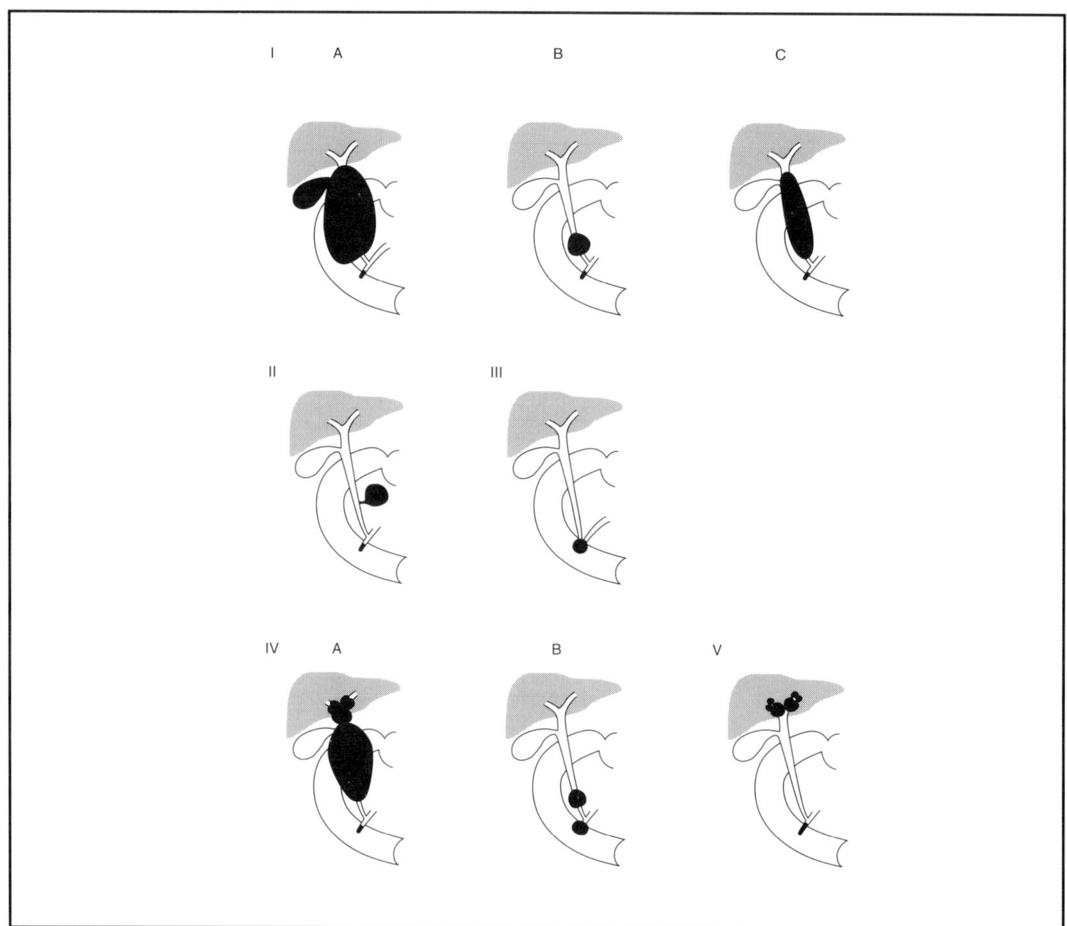

**Figure 2.17**
Schematic representation of the anatomic classification of Todani of choledochal cysts.

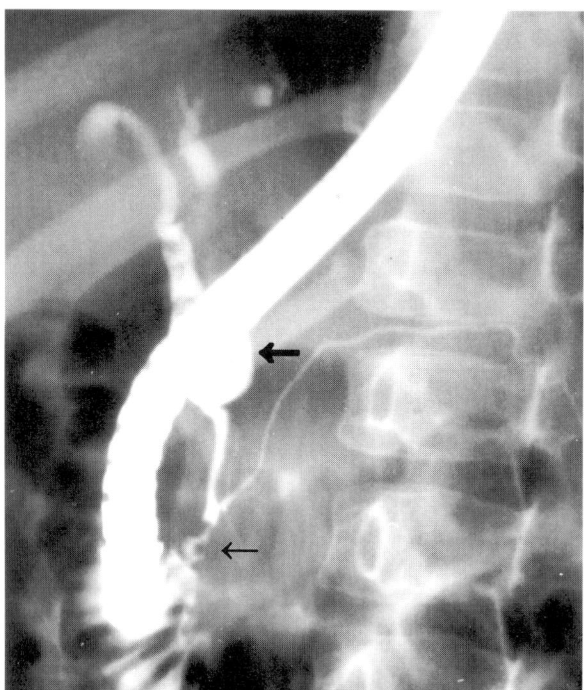

**Figure 2.18**
Choledochal cyst Type IA in a 7-year-old female. Long pancreaticobiliary union (↑). Normal pancreatic duct. Typical cyst dilatation of the common duct. Dilated cystic duct with stones (↑).

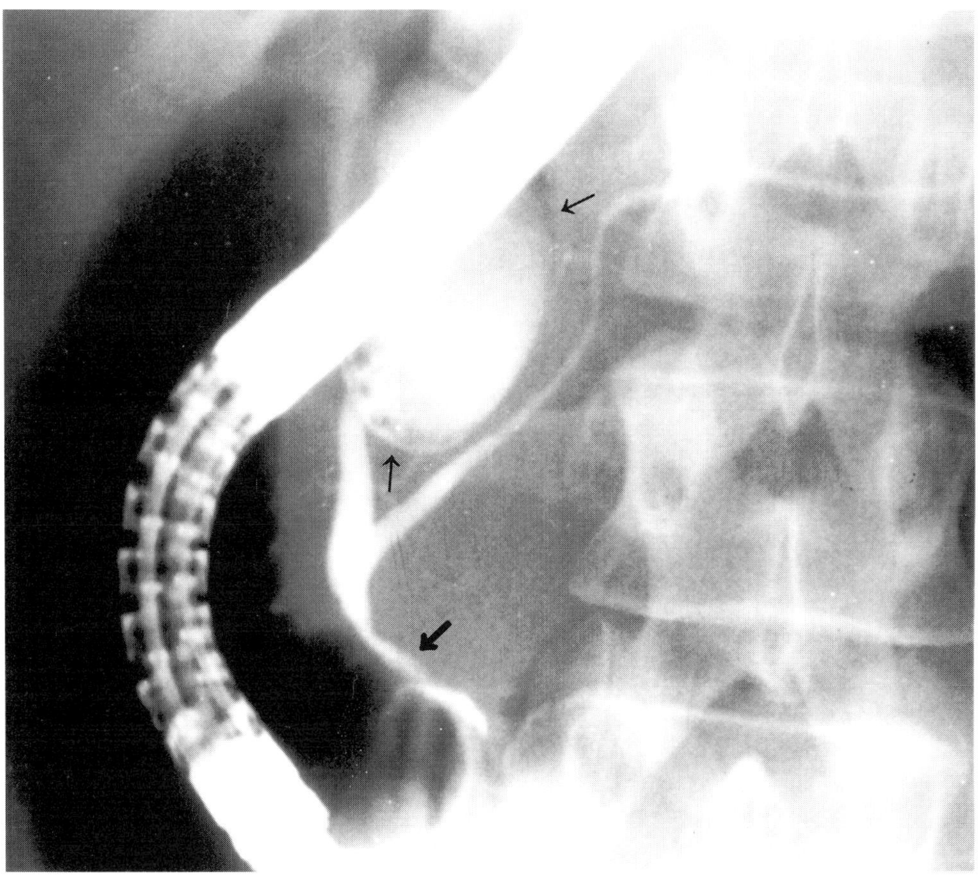

**Figure 2.19**
Choledochal cyst type IB in a 11-year-old female. Anomalous PB type union (↑).
Segmental common bile duct dilatation with cystic stones (↑).

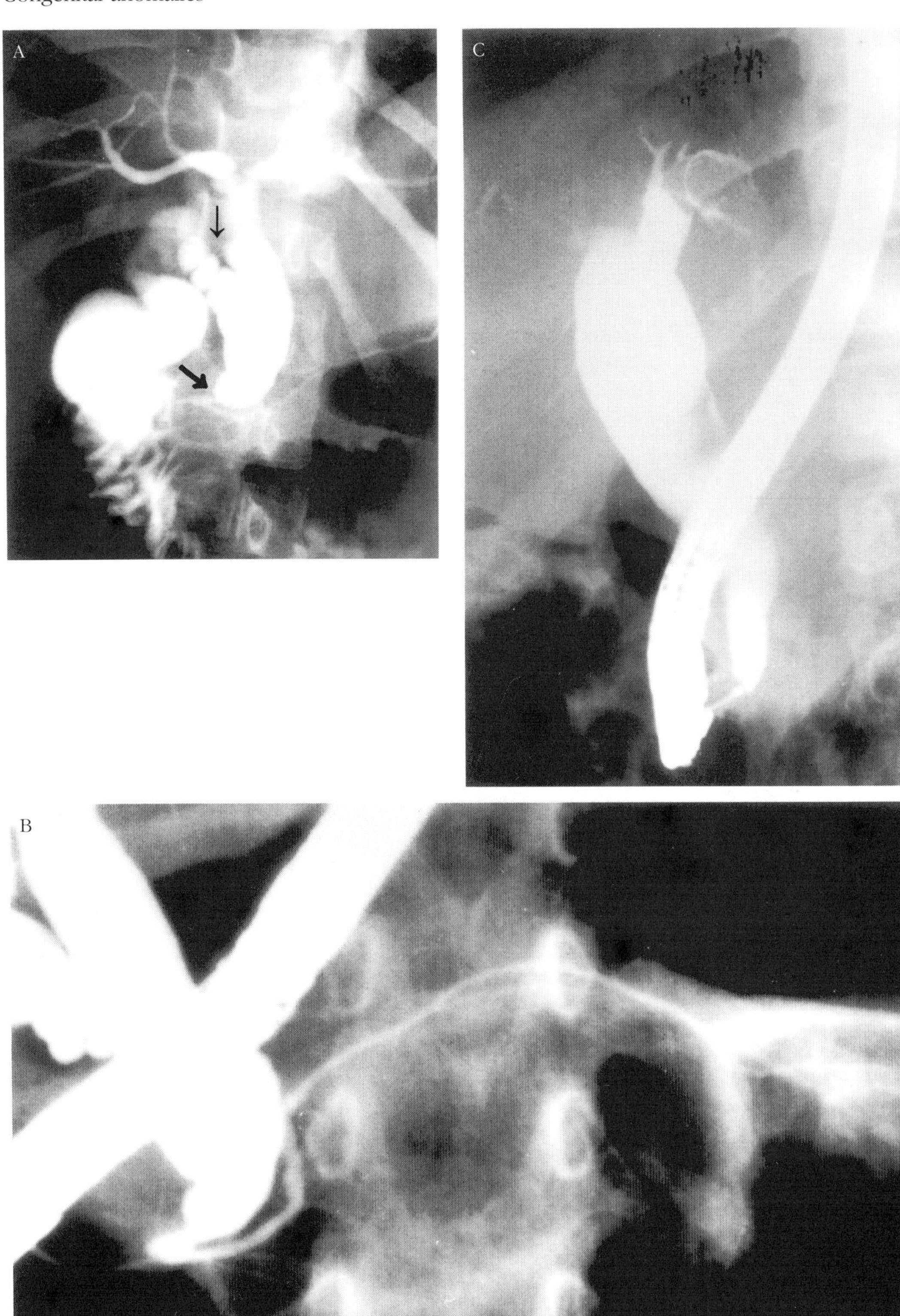

***Figure 2.20***
Choledochal cyst type IC. (A) A 9-year-old male with anomalous BP type union. Fusiform dilatation of the common duct. Dilated cystic duct (↑). Stricture at the distal common duct (↑). (B) After endoscopic sphincterotomy the common channel is wide open. The patient remained asymptomatic in the following 3 years. (C) Choledochal cyst type IC in a 7-year-old female. Fusiform dilatation of the entire common duct.

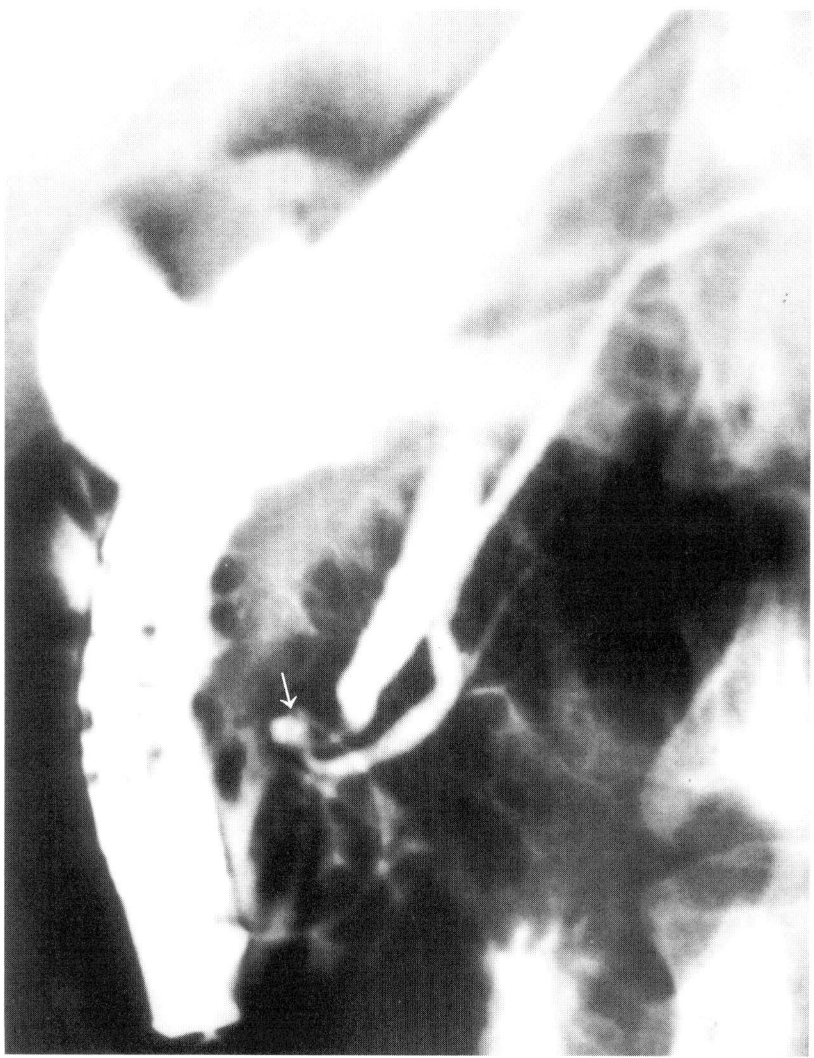

***Figure 2.21***
Choledochal cyst type III A in a 10-year-old male. Cystic dilatation of
the intraduodenal segment of the common duct (↑).

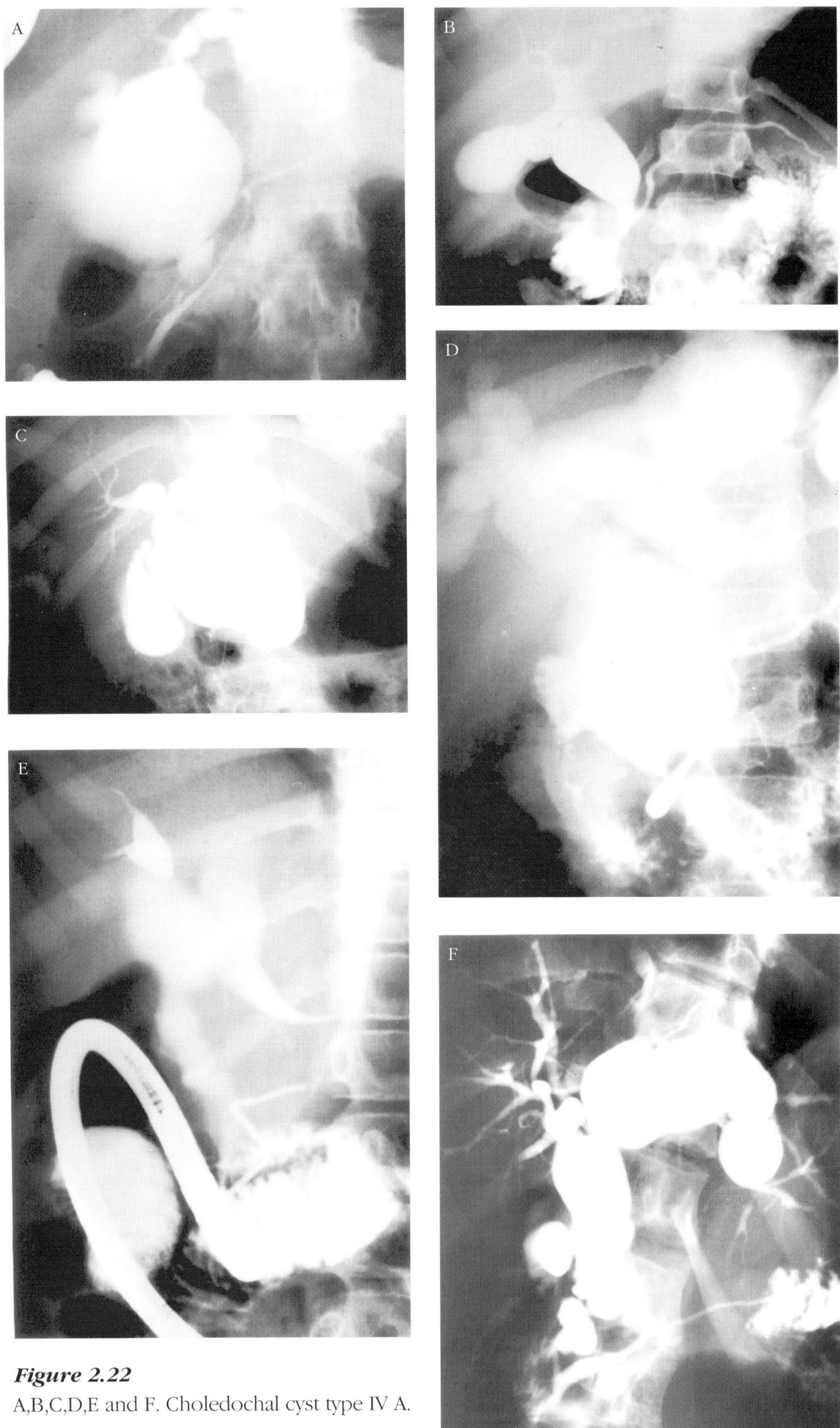

**Figure 2.22**
A,B,C,D,E and F. Choledochal cyst type IV A.

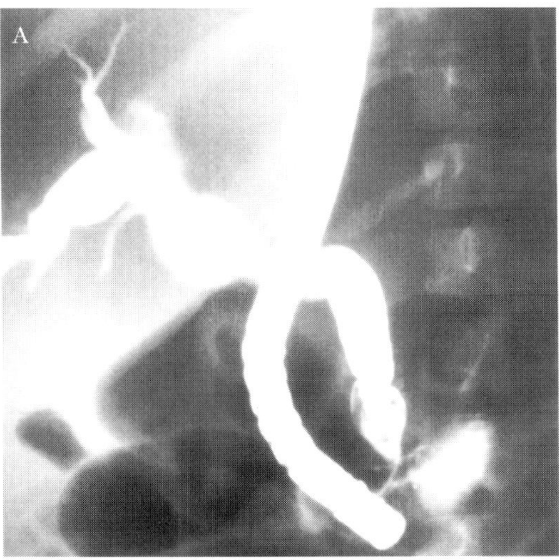 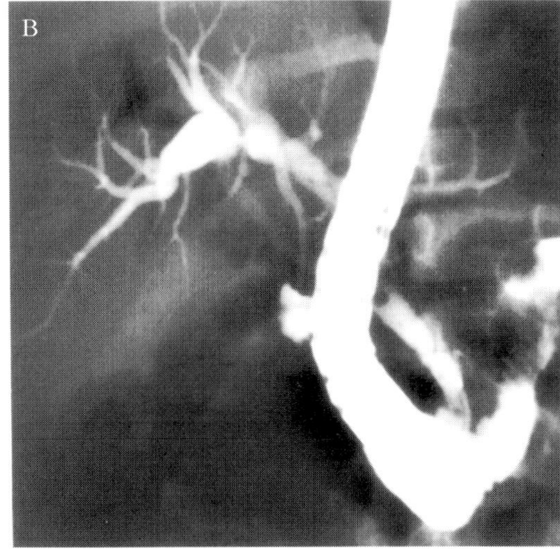

**Figure 2.23**

Choledochal cyst type IV B in a 2½-year-old female. (A) Cystic dilatation of the intrahepatic and extrahepatic ducts. Dilatation of the intraduodenal segment (choledochocele) with stones. (B) After endoscopic sphincterotomy and stone extraction the choledochocele disappear.

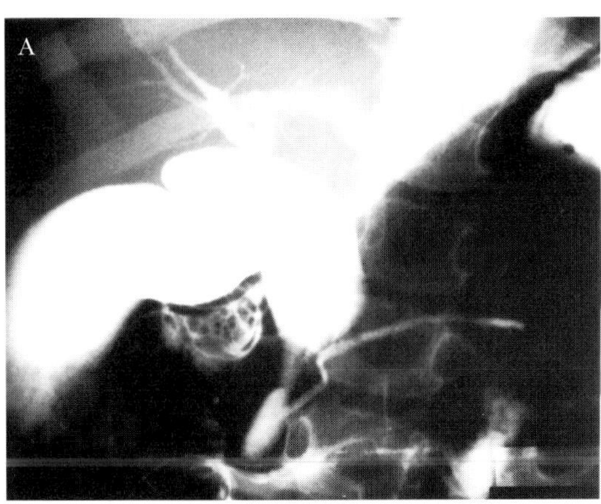 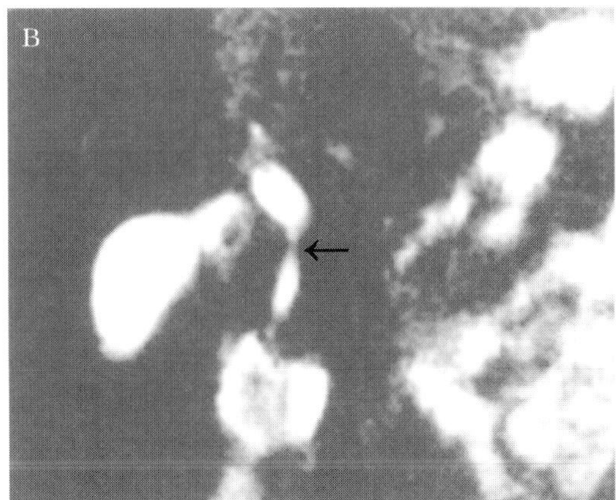

**Figure 2.24**

Choledochal cyst and magnetic resonance in a 4-year-old female. (A) Choledochal cyst type 1 C. Long PB type union. Irregular narrowing at the distal common duct. Diffuse dilatation of the common duct. Fusiform dilatation of the cystic duct. (B) Magnetic resonance. Narrowed common bile duct (↑) with a cystic dilatation above. No clear definition of the pancreaticobiliary junction.

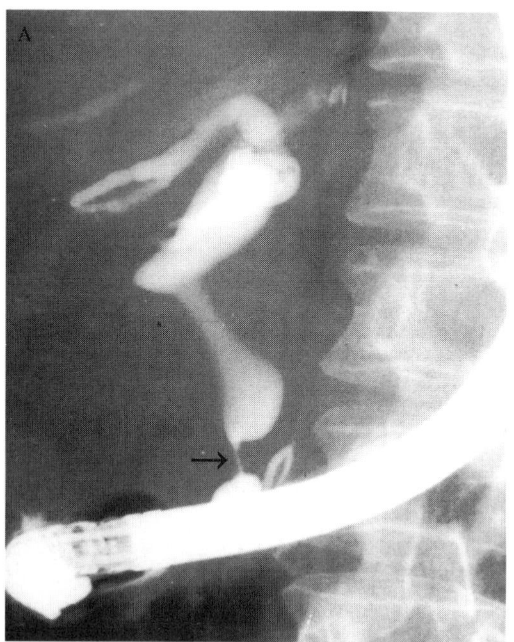
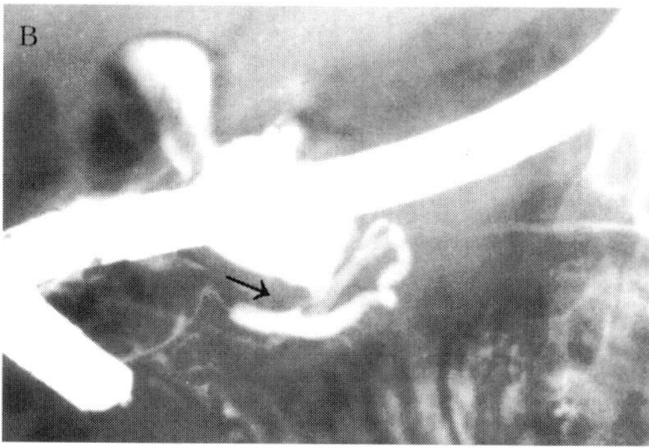

***Figure 2.25***
A and B. Choledochal cyst and distal bile duct stricture (↑).

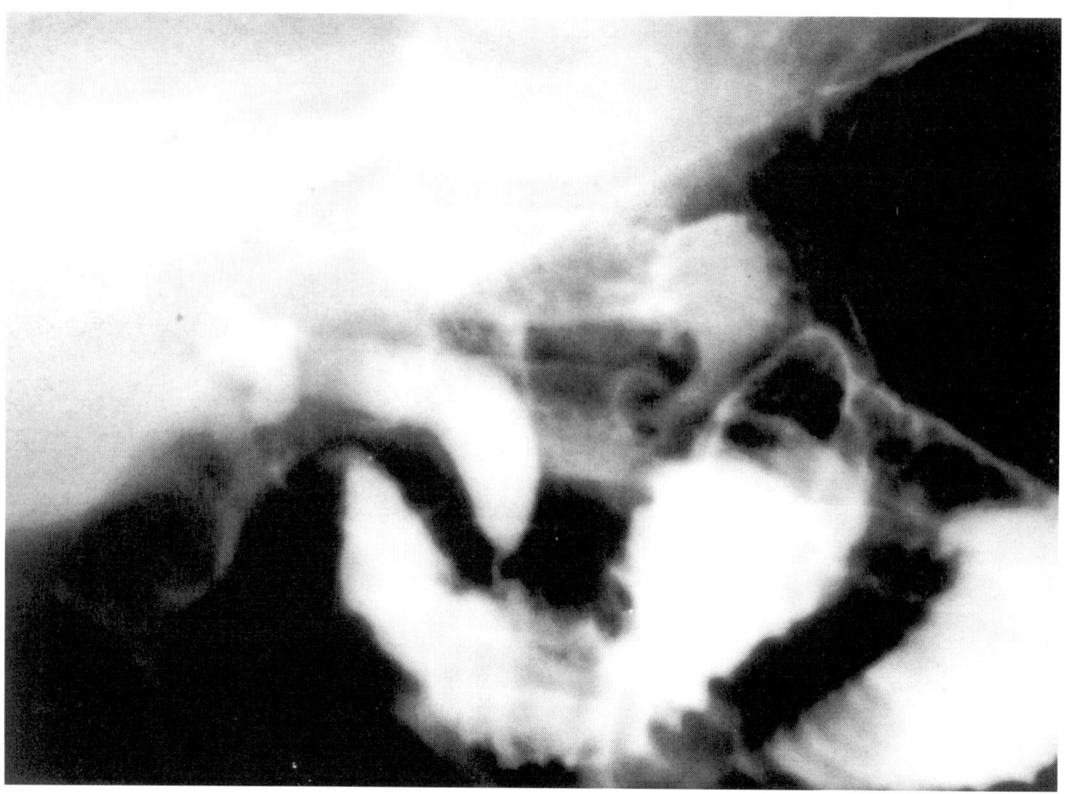

***Figure 2.26***
Choledochal cyst type IV A in a 29-day-old neonate with cholestasis. Cylindrical dilatation of the common bile duct and intrahepatic ducts. Stricture at the ductal bile duct.

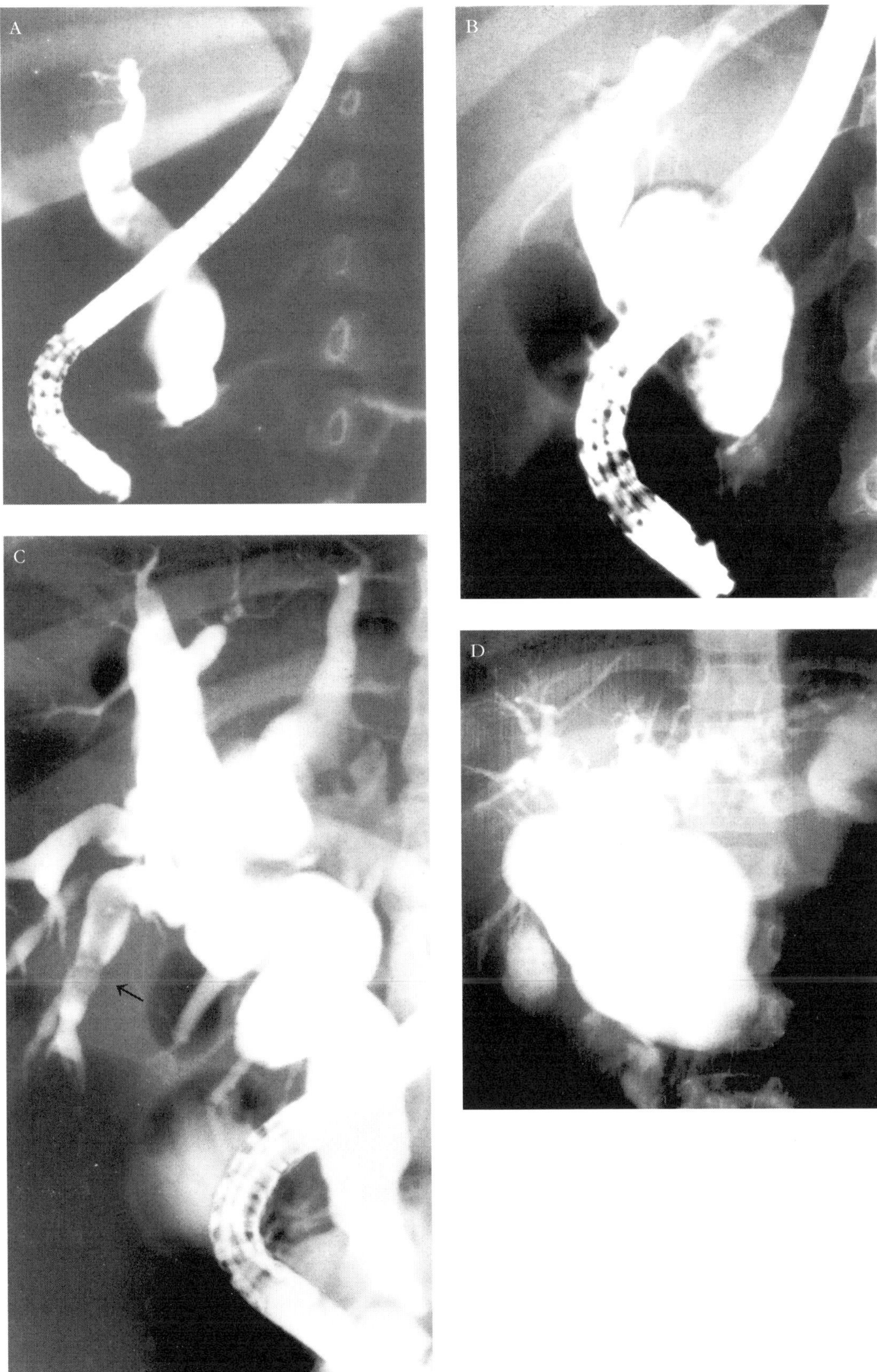

**Figure 2.27**
Choledochal cyst and lithiasis. (A) and (B) Cystolithiasis in the common bile duct in a type IC choledochal cyst. (C) Intrahepatic lithiasis (↑) in a type IV A choledochal cyst. (D) Gallstones in a type IV A choledochal cyst.

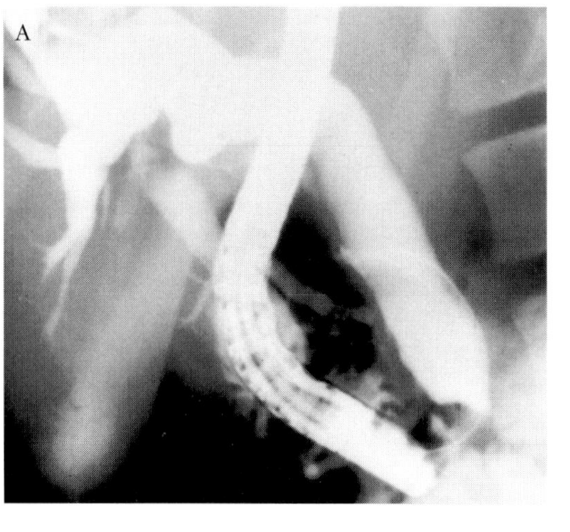
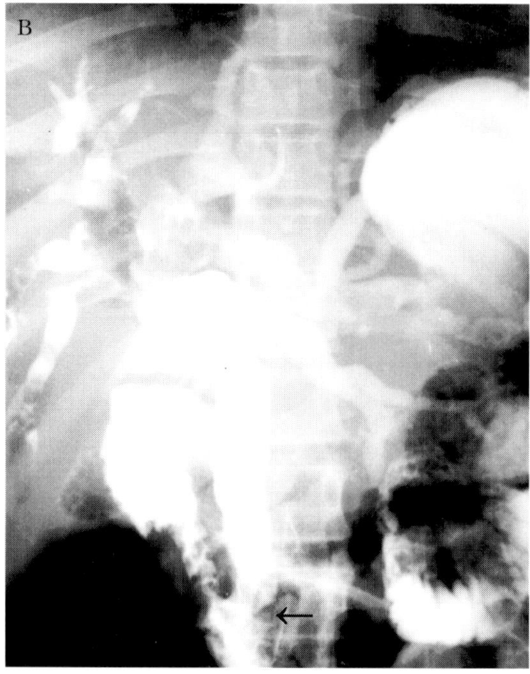

**Figure 2.28**

Choledochal cyst and endoscopic sphincterotomy in a 7-year-old female with type IV A choledochal cyst and recurrent cholestasis. (A) A sphincterotome is introduced into the common duct. (B) After sphincterotomy, air is visualized in the intrahepatic ducts; the distal common duct is wide open (↑).

# CHAPTER 3

# Acquired diseases

## Bile-plug syndrome

The bile-plug syndrome represents a correctable cause of obstruction of the extrahepatic bile ducts by bile sludge in patients without anatomic abnormalities of the biliary tract or hepatocellular lesions. Usually the syndrome occurs in infants with sepsis and acute dehydration (1). Clinically, bile-plug syndrome cannot be differentiated from biliary atresia. In the past, the diagnosis was made at exploratory laparotomy. Presently, the diagnosis is suggested by ultrasonographic findings which include dilatation of the biliary tree with sludge present within dilated ducts (2).

The inspissated material is usually removed surgically. Techniques include intraoperative irrigation of the biliary system with saline or a mucolytic agent, manual displacement of the plugs into the duodenum, and removal by sphincteroplasty (1–3). Others have reported spontaneous resolution after supportive therapy (2,4).

ERCP offers a diagnostic capability in this syndrome with therapeutic possibilities. In our experience with four jaundiced infants with normal liver biopsy and bile plugs in the parenchyma, abdominal ultrasound showed a dilated biliary tract. ERCP demonstrated a dilated common bile duct in all patients, two of whom had bile concrements (Fig. 3.1). The four patients cured after ERCP suggests that simple irrigation with contrast material may help remove concrements. (Fig. 3.2).

## Sclerosing cholangitis

Sclerosing cholangitis is a chronic hepatobiliary disease characterized by inflammation and obliterative fibrosis of the bile ducts, leading to biliary cirrhosis (5). In children, sclerosing cholangitis is associated with inflammatory bowel disease (5,6), histiocytosis X (7), immune deficiency states (8,9), and less frequently in patients with reticular cell sarcoma (10) and sickle cell anemia (11). However, sclerosing cholangitis has been reported in eight children with cholestasis without intestinal disease from the first week of life, followed by early cirrhosis (12).

In adults, 50–75% of patients with sclerosing cholangitis have concomitant inflammatory bowel disease (5). In children, this association is relatively uncommon (14%) suggesting that genetic and immunologic factors are the most important factors (13). The hypothesis that genetic factors may play a role in the etiology is supported by the finding of familial occurrence of sclerosing cholangitis both with or without associated ulcerative colitis (14) and by the report of neonatal sclerosing cholangitis in two siblings (15).

In children the disease begins insidiously, often making it difficult to diagnose. Some children may be seen initially with established cirrhosis. Therefore the diagnosis of sclerosing cholangitis can be established only by cholangiography. Radiologic examination by percutaneous cholecystography under ultrasound guidance carried out in eight children with cholestasis without intestinal disease (12) aged 8 months to 9 years, disclosed abnormal intrahepatic ducts with beaded appearance. The extrahepatic ducts were involved in six patients.

The disease in children is accurately diagnosed with ERCP as in adult patients (16). The cholangiogram will show pruning of the peripheral biliary tree and irregular areas of stenosis and ectasia reflecting the histopathological abnormalities manifested by inflammation and chronic fibrosis of the small and large biliary ducts. Liver biopsy is still used to obtain the diagnosis but changes seen on liver biopsy are not specific and at best only raise the possibility of sclerosing cholangitis (16). ERCP provides a more accurate and sensitive method of diagnosing sclerosing cholangitis (Fig. 3.3) and presently is the diagnostic procedure of choice (17).

Patients with ERCP findings of major ductal strictures in primary branches of large intrahepatic ducts or in the extrahepatic ducts are candidates for treatment with balloon dilatation (18,19) (Fig. 3.19). The goal is to relieve the obstruction in order to delay the progression to cirrhosis (20). Mechanical relief of obstruction through ERCP (19,21) or by percutaneous route (22) has produced immediate clinical and laboratory improvement. High-grade strictures can be dilated repeatedly, and the biliary tree can be cleared of stones or sludge. Because of the risk of cholangitis after stent placement, we prefer to dilate without placement of stents. Recently, we developed a new tapered hydrophilic balloon (Fig. 3.4) to dilate tight common duct strictures or hepatic duct strictures (Fig. 3.5), and to avoid small intrahepatic duct rupture (23). Brown *et al.* (24), studied five children with sclerosing cholangitis. Of these, three had dominant CBD strictures stented. Two patients demonstrated marked improvement of their liver function tests after stenting, and have been maintained with these devices for up to 1 year without complications. The third patient developed persistent abdominal pain after stent replacement, which resolved after stent removal 3 weeks later.

## Parasitic infestation

Hydatid disease, a parasitic infection with *Echinococcus granulosus*, involves the liver and has been confirmed by ERCP (25). Acute obstructive jaundice occurs in 5–17% of cases due to rupture of a liver cyst into the biliary tree either spontaneously or following surgery (26) and ERCP has proven to be a valuable technique for diagnosis of the disease and its complications (27). In the past, surgery was the only means of treatment. Recently, endoscopic sphincterotomy with removal of daughter cysts from the common bile duct has been successfully performed without complications (28,29).

Parasitic infestation with *Ascaris* can produce acute biliary obstruction with jaundice. The worm can be reliably demonstrated in both the bile ducts and gallbladder with the use of ultrasound and ERCP (Figs 3.6 and 3.7) (30). Treatment of biliary tract ascariasis has evolved from the direct removal of these worms through a surgical choledochotomy to an endoscopic removal from the common bile duct with a tripod basket (Figs 3.8 and 3.9) and other special instruments (31).

## Benign biliary strictures

Most of the benign biliary strictures are due to sclerosing cholangitis. Strictures may also result from operative injury, abdominal trauma, extrinsic compression from benign tumors or chronic pancreatitis, and congenital diaphragm or web (32). Primary stricture of the common hepatic duct has been described in a 3-year-old female with marked elevation of serum transaminases and without jaundice (33). We have seen a 14-year-old male with intermittent cholestasis and normal hepatic pathology since age 7 years, who had a web at the common hepatic duct demonstrated by ERCP that was initially treated with hydrostatic balloon dilation (Fig. 3.10). After a follow-up period of 4 years the patient developed another attack of acute cholangitis. Surgical excision of this web was curative.

## Malignant biliary strictures

Malignant strictures of the common bile duct are very uncommon in children. The diagnosis may be obtained by biopsy forceps of brush cytology through the therapeutic channel of the duodenoscope (34). Endoscopic biliary stenting has been used in adults with malignant strictures (35,36) for restoration of bile flow via placement of a stent across a stricture. Bickerstaff *et al.* (37) has successfully placed a stent in a 2-year-old boy for palliation of jaundice secondary to metastatic neuroblastoma. Guelrud *et al.* (38) reported the usefulness of ERCP for diagnosis and therapy in a 21-month-old child for stenting a malignant stricture in the common hepatic duct due to neuroblastoma (Fig. 3.11). A papillotomy was done and the stent was moved into position over a guidewire. Total bilirubin decreased from 29.6 mg/liter to 5.2 mg/liter after 3 days and chemotherapy could be started. Repeat ERCP after 4 months of chemotherapy showed disappearance of the compression and the biliary endoprosthesis was removed.

## Cholelithiasis and choledocholithiasis

The increased awareness of factors predisposing to cholelithiasis and the utilization of ultrasonography has led to the increasing diagnosis of cholelithiasis and common bile duct stones in children (39). Cholelithiasis is rare in childhood, and at the Mayo Clinic it represents 0.13% of all instances of cholelithiasis (40). Predisposing factors include chronic hemolysis (41), total parenteral nutrition with or without administration of furosemide (42,43). Terminal ileal pathology (44), maternal diabetes and pre-eclampsia (45), chronic idiopathic intestinal pseudo-obstruction (46), Down's syndrome (47), and biliary tract anomalies (48). However, 20–50% of gallstones in infants are thought to be idiopathic (39,40,49). Reports have been published on spontaneous resolution of cholelithiasis (50–52) and choledocholithiasis (53), and other studies emphasize the long-term complications of untreated cholelithiasis (41,42).

Ultrasonography is the method of choice for demonstration of cholelithiasis (41). Occasionally, ERCP may opacify the gallbladder and diagnose gallstones not seen by ultrasonography. Guelrud *et al.* (54) reported two young infants and two children with jaundice due to common bile duct stones (Fig. 3.12) in whom ultrasonography failed to show gallstones in one, but ERCP demonstrated gallstones in all four.

Choledocholithiasis occurs rarely in both infants and children (55). Conditions associated with the presence of stones include biliary tract malformations such as choledochal cyst, chronic liver disease, hemolysis and infection. The diagnostic approach is more difficult, and identification of the cause of obstruction by ultrasonography is often impossible. ERCP is the best technique in demonstrating common bile duct stones and is clearly superior to ultrasonography. In 10 jaundiced children with choledocholithiasis diagnosed by ERCP, ultrasonography demonstrated a common bile duct stone in only one patient (54).

Laparoscopic cholecystectomy is the treatment of choice in gallstone disease in adults. The major advantages of the procedure, compared with open cholecystectomy, are a shortened hospital stay, decreased post-operative pain, and shortened recovery period because of the lack of post-operative ileus (56). In children, the procedure has been reported in nine young patients with sickle hemoglobinopathies, ranging in age from 8.7 to 19.8 years (57). The mean post-operative hospital stay was 1.6 days, and no complications resulted from the procedure. Intraoperative cholangiograms were possible in only five of the nine patients. If a common bile duct stone is found during laparoscopic cholecystectomy, the procedure should be converted to an open cholecystectomy. In adults, if choledocholithiasis is suspected, ERCP with endoscopic sphincterotomy and stone removal has been performed before laparoscopic cholecystectomy (58). The same approach can be advocated for children and is our current practice. If no common bile duct stone is found during ERCP in a patient with known gallstones, the endoscopist may elect to perform prophylactic or protective sphincterotomy, enabling more elective scheduling of the subsequent cholecystectomy. The risk of added complications from sphincterotomy must be balanced against the inconvenience of urgent cholecystectomy and the potential morbidity of repeat common bile duct stone impaction or open cholecystectomy.

Endoscopic sphincterotomy is the treatment of choice in the management of retained and recurrent bile duct stones for adult patients (59) with a success rate of up to 96% (60). In children, sphincterotomy with common bile duct stone removal has been performed in infants as young as 2 months old (80). Man and Spitz (62) performed a sphincterotomy with clearing of the duct by dragging out debris with a Fogarty catheter in a 3-year-old child. Buckley and Connon (63) successfully performed endoscopic sphincterotomy in five children and achieved common bile duct stone removal without significant complications. Guelrud *et al.* (54) treated six jaundiced children with choledocholithiasis who have had the gallbladder removed for gallstones, by endoscopic sphincterotomy and stone extraction using a Dormia basket (Fig. 3.13) or Fogarty balloons without complications. Recently, a 6-month-old jaundiced infant with choledocholithiasis and sepsis (Fig. 3.14) was successfully treated by endoscopic sphincterotomy and stone retrieval without complications (61). Brown *et al.* (24) performed sphincterotomy in five children with common bile duct stones and one with intrahepatic duct stones without complications.

Most infants with asymptomatic gallstones and no factors that would make them susceptible to stone formation can be managed conservatively (48,50–53). However, larger stones are less likely to resolve, whereas smaller stones, sludge and mucus should be able to pass in response to oral feeding without symptoms or complications. The larger the stone, the greater the probability that obstruction will occur. It appears that an aggressive approach is not warranted in the asymptomatic infant. Surgery, radiology or endoscopy intervention should be reserved for symptomatic patients or those with underlying lithogenic disorders.

A combined endoscopic sphincterotomy and laparoscopic cholecystectomy has been successfully reported in adults (58) and in children (64) (Fig. 3.15). An advantage of this approach is that if endoscopic removal of a common duct stone is not possible, it allows the surgeon to proceed directly to open common duct exploration avoiding additional operative procedure. On the contrary, if endoscopic removal of common duct stones is possible, the advantage inherent to laparoscopic cholecystectomy will be maintained. Although the combined procedure seems to be safe. Additional experience has to be awaited so that the true advantages, limitations and complications of this approach can be placed into clinical perspective.

## Liver transplantation

In patients whose liver is transplanted, the integrity of the anastomosis can be studied (Fig. 3.16). Whereas ERCP is not feasible in patients with a choledochojejunostomy after transplantation, it is an alternative to percutaneous transhepatic cholangiography in patients with choledochoduodenostomy and choledochocholedochostomy and is the procedure of choice in patients with coagulopathy when the biliary tree must be imaged. When a stricture is found (65–67), the area may be dilated (18,68) and a stent may be placed for a limited period of time (19); in the same manner bile leaks may be found (Fig. 3.17) (65,67,69) and can be treated by endoscopic sphincterotomy or with stent placement (70,71).

## Acquired immunodeficiency syndrome

Biliary tract involvement in immunodeficiency syndrome may at times be difficult to distinguish from hepatic parenchymal disease. Common bile duct stones, cholecystitis, sclerosing cholangitis, strictures, papillitis, papillary stenosis, and infections with cytomegalovirus and cryptosporidium have been reported in adults (72–75). Relatively little has been published regarding biliary involvement in children with AIDS (76–78). Affected children usually complain of abdominal pain and jaundice. Children with cytomegalovirus often have evidence of cholestasis even in the absence of symptoms, supporting a role for cytomegalovirus in the AIDS cholangiopathy (79). An extrahepatic cause for jaundice is suggested on ultrasonography or CT by the presence of dilated ducts or other biliary abnormalities. Further evaluation may include ERCP which provides definitive diagnosis with potential for therapeutic intervention. In cases of papillary stenosis (Fig. 3.18), endoscopic sphincterotomy can safely be performed. Biliary fluid and biopsy specimens from the ampulla of Vater should be taken and examined for the presence of viruses, protozoa or neoplastic cells. Recently, Naon *et al.* (77), performed endoscopic sphincterotomy and common bile duct dilatation in two children with papillary stenosis and common duct stricture resulting in a significant improvement of pain. No microorganisms were isolated from biliary fluid obtained during the procedure. Yabut *et al.* (78) reported four children with HIV infection in whom ERCP was performed. Three patients had sclerosing cholangitis. Cytomegalovirus infection was demonstrated in two patients. One child had invasive cryptosporidium in the biopsies of the papilla of Vater. Two patients had associated papillary stenosis. There were no complications.

## References


1. Bernstein J, Braylan R, Brough AJ. Bile-plug syndrome: a correctable cause of obstructive jaundice in infants. *Pediatrics* 1969; **43:** 273–6.
2. Mahr MA, Hugosson C, Nazer HM, *et al.* Bile-plug syndrome. *Pediatr Radiol* 1988; **19:** 61–4.
3. Brown DM. Bile plug syndrome: successful management with a mucolytic agent. *J Pediatr Surg* 1990; **25:** 351–2.
4. Sty JR, Wells RG, Schroeder BA. Comparative imaging. Bile-plug syndrome. *Clin Nucl Med* 1987; **12:** 489–90.
5. Weisner RH, Grambsch PM, Dickson ER, *et al.* Primary sclerosing cholangitis: natural history, prognostic factors and survival analysis. *Hepatology* 1989; **10:** 430–6.
6. Classen M, Golze H, Richter HJ, *et al.* Primary sclerosing cholangitis in children. *J Pediatr Gastroenterol Nutr* 1987; **6:** 197–202.
7. Leblanc A, Hadchouel M, Jehan P, *et al.* Obstructive jaundice in children with histiocytosis X. *Gastroenterology* 1981; **80:** 134–9.
8. Record CO, Eddelston AL, Shilkin KB, *et al.* Intrahepatic sclerosing cholangitis associated with familial immunodeficiency syndrome. *Lancet* 1973; **2:** 18–20.
9. DiPalma JA, Strobel CT, Farrow JG. Primary sclerosing cholangitis associated with hyperimmunoglobulin M immunodeficiency (dysgammablobulinemia). *Gastroenterology* 1986; **91:** 464–8.
10. Alpert LI, Jindrak K. Idiopathic retroperitoneal fibrosis and sclerosing cholangitis associated with a reticulum cell sarcoma. *Gastroenterology* 1972; **62:** 111–7.

11. Werlin LS, Glicklich M, Jona J, *et al.* Sclerosing cholangitis in childhood. *J Pediatr* 1980; **96:** 433–5.

12. Amedee-Manesme O, Bernard O, Brunelle F, Hadchouel M, Polonovski C, Baudon JJ, Beguet P, Alagille D. Sclerosing cholangitis with neonatal onset. *J Pediatr* 1987; **111:** 225–9.

13. Debray D, Pariente D, Urroas E, *et al.* Sclerosing cholangitis in children. *J Pediatr* 1994; **124:** 49–56.

14. Quigly EM, La Russo NF, Ludwig E. Familial occurrence of primary sclerosing cholangitis and ulcerative colitis. *Gastroenterology* 1983; **85:** 1160–5.

15. Baker AJ, Portmann B, Westby D, *et al.* Neonatal sclerosing cholangitis in two siblings: a category of progressive intrahepatic cholestasis. *J Pediatr Gastroenterol Nutr* 1993; **17:** 317–22.

16. Ludwing J, Mac Carty RL, La Russo NF, Krom RA, Wiesner RH. Intrahepatic cholangiectasis and large duct obstruction in primary sclerosing cholangitis. *Hepatology* 1986; **6:** 560–8.

17. MacCarty RL, LaRusso NF, Wiesner RH, Ludwing J. Primary sclerosing cholangitis: findings in cholangiography and pancreatography. *Radiology* 1983; **49:** 39–44.

18. Siegel JH, Guelrud M. Endoscopic cholangiopancreatoplasty: hydrostatic balloon dilation in the bile duct and pancreas. *Gastrointest Endosc* 1983; **29:** 99–103.

19. Johnson GK, Geenen JE, Venu RP, Schmalz MJ, Hogan WJ. Endoscopic treatment of biliary tract strictures in sclerosing cholangitis: a larger series and recommendations for treatment. *Gastrointest Endosc* 1991; **37:** 38–43.

20. Lee JG, Schutz SM, England RE, Leung JW, Cotton PB. Endoscopic therapy of sclerosing cholangitis. *Hepatology* 1995; **21:** 661–7.

21. Stoker J, Lameris JS, Robben SG, *et al.* Primary sclerosing cholangitis in a child treated by non-surgical balloon dilatation and stenting. *J Pediatr Gastroenterol Nutr* 1993; **17:** 303–6.

22. Skolkin MD, Alspaugh JP, Casarella WU, *et al.* Sclerosing cholangitis: palliation with percutaneous cholangioplasty. *Radiology* 1989; **170:** 199–206.

23. Guelrud M, Mendoza S, Gelrud A. A tapered balloon with hydrophilic coating to dilate difficult hilar biliary strictures. *Gastrointest Endosc* 1995; **41:** 246–9.

24. Brown KO, Golschmiedt M. Endoscopic therapy of biliary and pancreatic disorders in children. *Endoscopy* 1994; **26:** 719–23.

25. Cottone M, Amuso M, Cotton PB. Endoscopic retrograde cholangiography in hepatic hydatid disease. *Br J Surg* 1978; **65:** 107–8.

26. Katan YB. Intrabiliary rupture of hydatid cyst of the liver. *Br J Surg* 1975; **62:** 885–90.

27. Vicente VFM, Garcia EM, Marco MAS. Endoscopic retrograde cholangiography and complicated hepatic hydatid cyst in the biliary tract. *Endoscopy* 1984; **16:** 124–6.

28. Al Karawi MA, Mohamed AE, Yassawy I. Non-surgical endoscopic trans-papillary treatment of ruptured *Echinococcus* liver cyst obstructing the biliary tree. *Endoscopy* 1987; **19:** 81–3.

29. Vignote ML, Mino G, De La Mata M, Dios JF, Gomez F. Endoscopic sphincterotomy in hepatic hydatid disease open to the biliary tree. *Br J Surg* 1990; **77:** 30–1.

30. Van Der Spuy S. Endoscopic retrograde cholangiopancreatography (ERCP) in children. *Endoscopy* 1978; **10:** 173–5.

31. Guelrud M. Endoscopic retrograde cholangiopancreatography in the infant. In: Barkin J, O'Phelan, eds. *Advanced Therapeutic Endoscopy.* New York: Raven Press, 1990: 335–4.

32. Melmen RE, Nahra K. Congenital diaphragm of the common hepatic duct. *Br J Radiol* 1966; **39:** 392–4.

33. Chapoy PR, Kendall RS, Fonkalsrud E, Ament ME. Congenital stricture of the common hepatic duct: an unusual case without jaundice. *Gastroenterology* 1981; **80:** 380–3.

34. Rustgi AK, Kelsey PB, Guelrud M, Saini S, Schapiro RH. Malignant tumors of the bile ducts: diagnosis by biopsy during endoscopic cannulation. *Gastrointest Endosc* 1989; **35:** 248–51.

35. Sohendra N, Grimm H, Berger B, Nam VC. Malignant jaundice: results of diagnostic and therapeutic endoscopy. *World J Surg* 1989; **13:** 171–7.

36. Soehendra N, Reynders-Frederix V. Palliative bile duct drainage. A new endoscopic method of introducing a transpapillary drain. *Endoscopy* 1980; **12:** 8–11.

37. Bickerstaff KI, Britton BJ, Gough MH. Endoscopic palliation of malignant biliary obstruction in a child. *Br J Surg* 1989; **76:** 1092–3.

38. Guelrud M, Mendoza S, Zager A, Noguera C. Biliary stenting in an infant with malignant obstructive jaundice. *Gastrointest Endosc* 1989; **35:** 259–61.

39. Garel L, Lallemand D, Montagne JP, Forel F, Sauvegrain J. The changing aspects of cholelithiasis in children through a sonographic study. *Pediatr Radiol* 1981; **11:** 75–9.

40. Brenner RW, Stewart CF. Cholecystitis in children. *Rev Surg* 1964; **21:** 327–31.

41. Brill PW, Winchester P, Rosen MS. Neonatal cholelithiasis. *Pediatr Radiol* 1982; **12:** 285–8.

42. Whitington PF, Black DD. Cholelithiasis in premature infants treated with parenteral nutrition and furosemide. *J Pediatr* 1980; **97:** 647–9.

43. King DR, Ginn-Pease ME, Lloyd TV, *et al.* Parenteral nutrition with associated cholelithiasis. Another iatrogenic disease of infants and children. *J Pediatr Surg* 1987; **22:** 593–6.

44. Pellerin D, Bertin P, Nihoul-Fekete A, *et al.* Cholelithiasis and ileal pathology in childhood. *J Pediatr Surg* 1975; **10:** 35–41.

45. Auni EF, Matos C, Gansbeke D, *et al.* Atypical gallbladder content in neonates: ultrasonic demonstration. *Ann Radiol* 1986; **29:** 267–73.

46. Shimotake T, Iwai N, Yanagihara J, Tokiwa K, Fushiki S. Biliary tract complications in patients with hypoganglionosis and chronic idiopathic intestinal pseudoobstruction syndrome. *J Pediatr Surg* 1993; **28:** 189–92.

47. Aughton DJ, Gibson P, Cacciarelli A. Cholelithiasis in infants with Down syndrome. Three cases and literature review. *Clin Pediatr* 1992; **11:** 650–2.

48. Lilly JR. Common bile duct calculi in infants and children. *J Pediatr Surg* 1980; **15:** 577–80.

49. St-Vil D, Yazbeck S, Luks FI, Hancock BJ, Filiatrault D, Youssef S. Cholelithiasis in newborns and infants. *J Pediatr Surg* 1992; **10:** 1305–7.

50. Keller MS, Markle BM, Laffey PA, *et al.* Spontaneous resolution of cholelithiasis in infants. *Radiology* 1985; **157:** 345–8.

51. Nabil NJ, Anderson KD, Eichelberger M, *et al.* Cholelithiasis in infancy: resolution of gallstones in three of four infants. *J Pediatr Surg* 1986; **21:** 567–9.

52. Schrimer WJ, Grisoni ER, Gauderer MWL. The spectrum of cholelithiasis in the first year of life. *J Pediatr Surg* 1989; **24:** 1064–7.

53. Holgersen LO, Stolar C, Berdon WE, Hilfer C, Levy JS. Therapeutic and diagnostic implications of acquired choledochal obstruction in infancy: spontaneous resolution in three infants. *J Pediatr Surg* 1990; **25:** 1027–9.

54. Guelrud M, Mendoza S, Jaen D, Plaz J, Machuca J, Torres P. ERCP and endoscopic sphincterotomy in infants and children with jaundice due to common bile duct stones. *Gastrointest Endosc* 1992; **38:** 450–3.

55. Shaw PJ, Spitz L, Watson JG. Extrahepatic biliary obstruction due to stone. *Arch Dis Child* 1984; **59:** 896–7.

56. Dubois F, Icard P, Berthelot G, Levard H. Celioscopic cholecystectomy. *Ann Surg* 1990; **211:** 60–2.

57. Ware RE, Kinney TR, Casey JR, Pappas TN, Meyers WC. Laparoscopic cholecystectomy in young patients with sickle hemoglobinopathies. *J Pediatr* 1992; **120:** 58–61.

58. Aliperti G, Edmundowicz SA, Soper NJ, Combined endoscopic sphincterotomy and laparoscopic cholecystectomy in patients with choledocholithiasis and cholecystolithiasis. *Ann Intern Med* 1991; **115:** 783–4.

59. Geenen JE, Vennes JA, Silvis SE. Resume of seminar on endoscopic retrograde sphincterotomy. *Gastrointest Endosc* 1981; **27:** 31–8.

60. Cotton PB. Endoscopic management of bile duct stones; (apples and oranges). *Gut* 1984; **25:** 587–97.

61. Guelrud M, Daoud G, Mendoza S, *et al.* Endoscopic sphincterotomy in a 6-month-old infant with choledocholithiasis and double gallbladder. *Am J Gastroenterol* 1994; **89:** 1587–9.

62. Man DW, Spitz L. Choledocholithiasis in infancy. *J Ped Surg* 1985; **20:** 65–8.

63. Buckley A, Connon JJ. The role of ERCP in children and adolescents. *Gastrointest Endosc* 1990; **36:** 369–72.

64. Guelrud M, Zambrano V, Jaen D, *et al.* Endoscopic sphincterotomy and laparoscopic cholecystectomy in a jaundiced infant. *Gastrointest Endosc* 1994; **40:** 99–102.

65. Putnam PE, Kocoshis SA, Orenstein SR, Schade RR. Pediatric endoscopic retrograde cholangiopancreatography. *Am J Gastroenterol* 1991; **86:** 824–30.

66. Evans RA, Raby ND, O'Grady JG, *et al.* Biliary complications following orthotopic liver transplantation. *Clin Radiol* 1990; **41:** 190–4.

67. Peclet MH, Ryckman FC, Pedersen SH, *et al.* The spectrum of bile duct complications in pediatric liver transplantation. *J Pediatr Surg* 1994; **29:** 214–19.

68. Geenen DJ, Geenen JE, Hogan WJ, *et al.* Endoscopic therapy for benign bile duct strictures. *Gastrointest Endosc* 1989; **35:** 367–1.

69. Dominguez R, Young LW, Ledesma-Medina J, *et al.* Pediatric liver transplantation. Part II. Diagnostic imaging in postoperative management. *Radiology* 1985; **157:** 339–44.

70. Osorio RW, Freise CE, Stock PG, *et al.* Nonoperative management of biliary leaks after orthotopic liver transplantation. *Transplantation* 1993; **55:** 1074–7.

71. Porcheron, J, Boillot O, Ponchon T, *et al.* Treatments of biliary fistulas following the removal of a Kehr tube after orthotopic liver transplantation. *Ann Chir* 1994; **48:** 441–5.

72. Pitlik SD, Fainstein V, Rios A, *et al.* Cryptosporidial cholecystitis. *N Engl J Med* 1983; **308:** 1967.

73. Schneiderman DJ, Cello JP, Laing FC. Papillary stenosis and sclerosing cholangitis in the acquired immunodeficiency syndrome. *Ann Intern Med* 1987; **106:** 546–9.

74. Bonacini M. Hepatobiliary complications in patients with human immunodeficiency virus infection. *Am J Med* 1992; **92:** 404–11.

75. Bouche H, Housset C, Dumont JL, *et al.* AIDS-related cholangitis: diagnostic features and course in 15 patients. *J Hepatol* 1993; **17:** 34–9.

76. Miller TL, Winter HS, Luginbuhl LM, *et al.* Pancreatitis in pediatric human immunodeficiency virus infection. *J Pediatr* 1992; **120:** 223–7.

77. Naon H, Shelton M, Thomas D, *et al.* Retrograde-cholangio-pancreatic videoendoscopy (ERCP) findings in pediatric patients with acquired immune deficiency syndrome (AIDS). *Gastrointest Endosc* 1995; **41:** A340.

78. Yabut B, Werlin SL, Havens P, *et al.* Endoscopic retrograde cholangiopancreatography in children with HIV infection. *J Pediatr Gastroenterol Nutr* 1996; **23:** 624–7.

79. Jacobson MA, Cello JP, Sande MS. Cholestasis and disseminated cytomegalovirus disease in patients with acquired immunodeficiency syndrome. *Am J Med* 1988; **84:** 218–24.

80. Wilkinson ML, Clayton PT. Sphincterotomy for jaundice in a neonate. *J Pediatr Gastroenterol Nutr* 1996; **23:** 507–9.

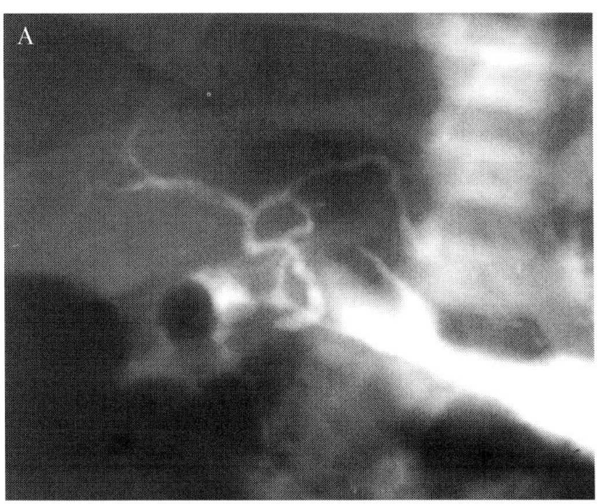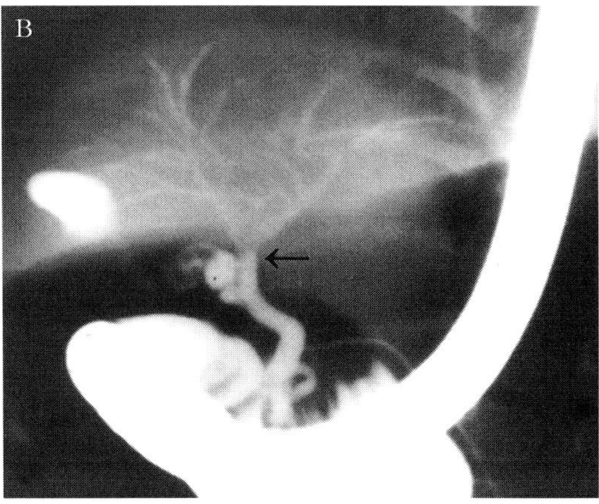

***Figure 3.1***

(A) Bile-plug syndrome in a 21-day-old female jaundiced neonate. Dilatation of the extrahepatic biliary tree. Patient improved after ERCP. (B) Bile-plug syndrome in a 45-day-old young infant with cholestasis. Dilatation of the extrahepatic biliary tree. Concrements in the main hepatic duct (↑) and in the gallbladder. Jaundice disappeared after ERCP.

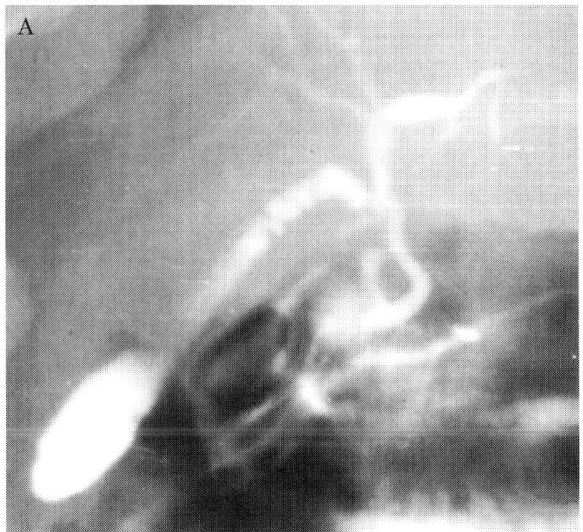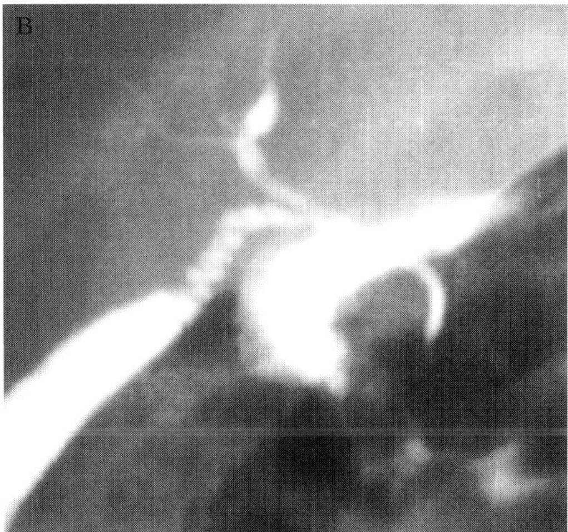

***Figure 3.2***

(A) Bile-plug syndrome in a 2-month-old jaundiced infant. Dilatation of the extrahepatic biliary tract. Patient improved after ERCP. (B) Same patient 4 months later. Normal extrahepatic biliary tract.

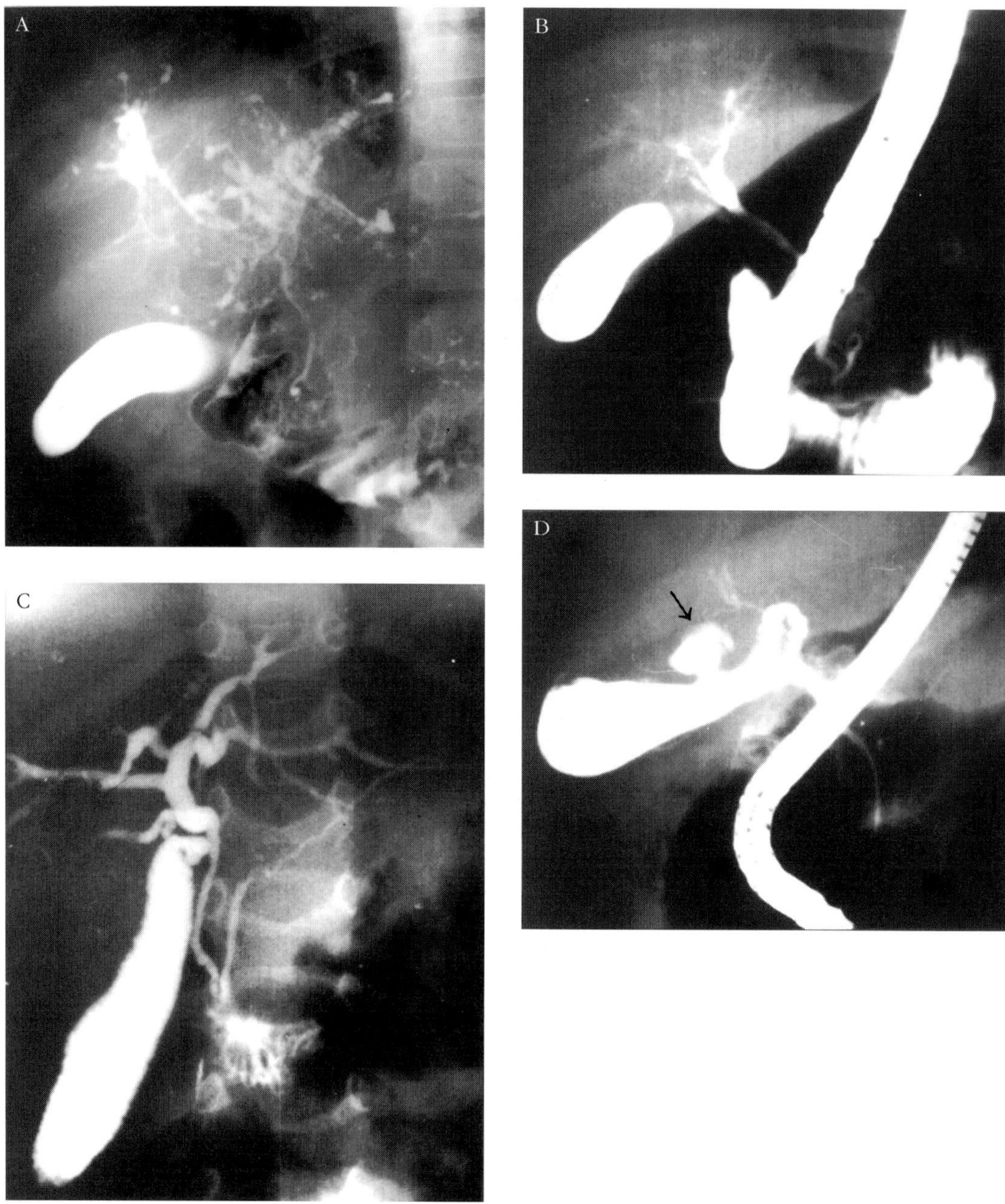

**Figure 3.3**
Sclerosing cholangitis. ERCP shows pruning of the peripheral biliary tree and irregular areas of stenosis and ectasia. (A) A 12-year-old female with ulcerative colitis. (B) A 2-month-old male without inflammatory bowel disease. (C) A 3-year-old male without inflammatory disease. (D) A 5-year-old male without inflammatory disease. A gallbladder diverticulum is visualized (↑).

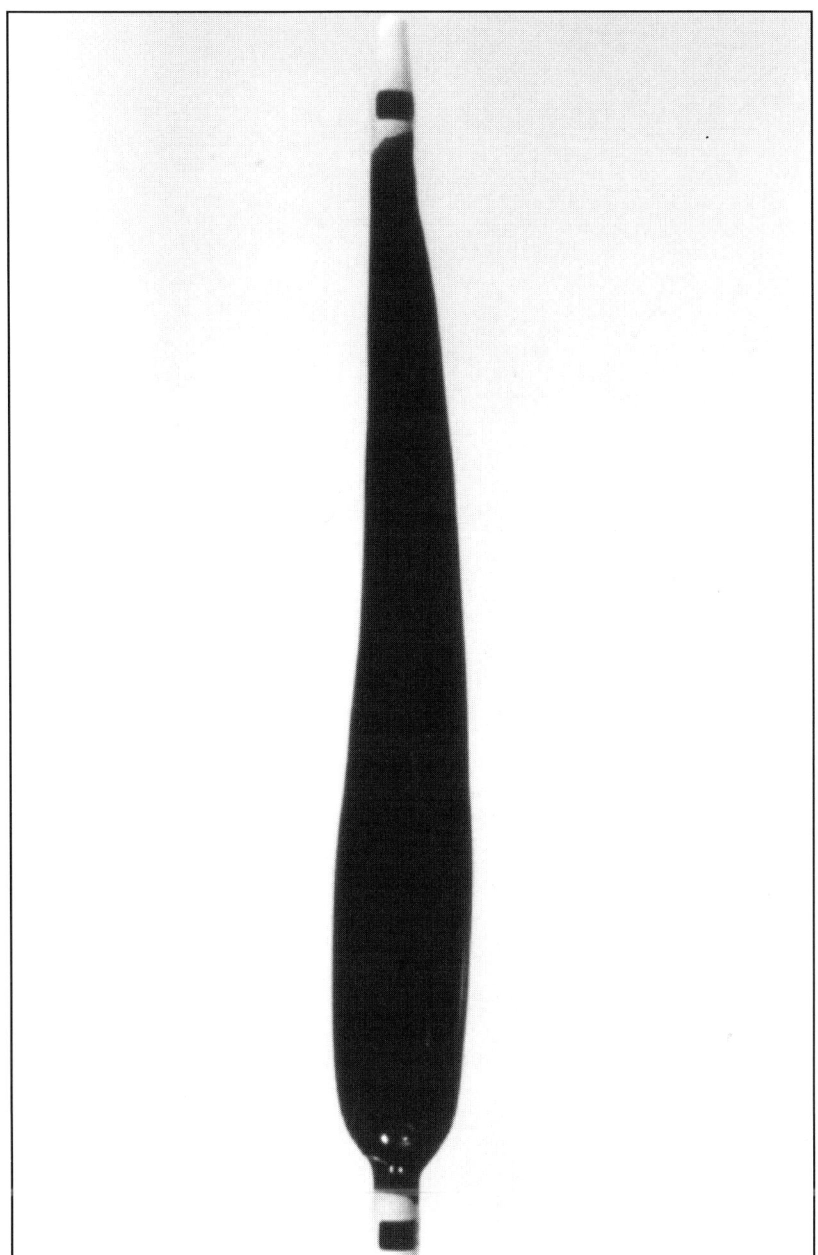

***Figure 3.4***
A tapered hydrophilic balloon fully inflated used to dilate hepatic duct strictures and to avoid rupture of the small intrahepatic ducts.

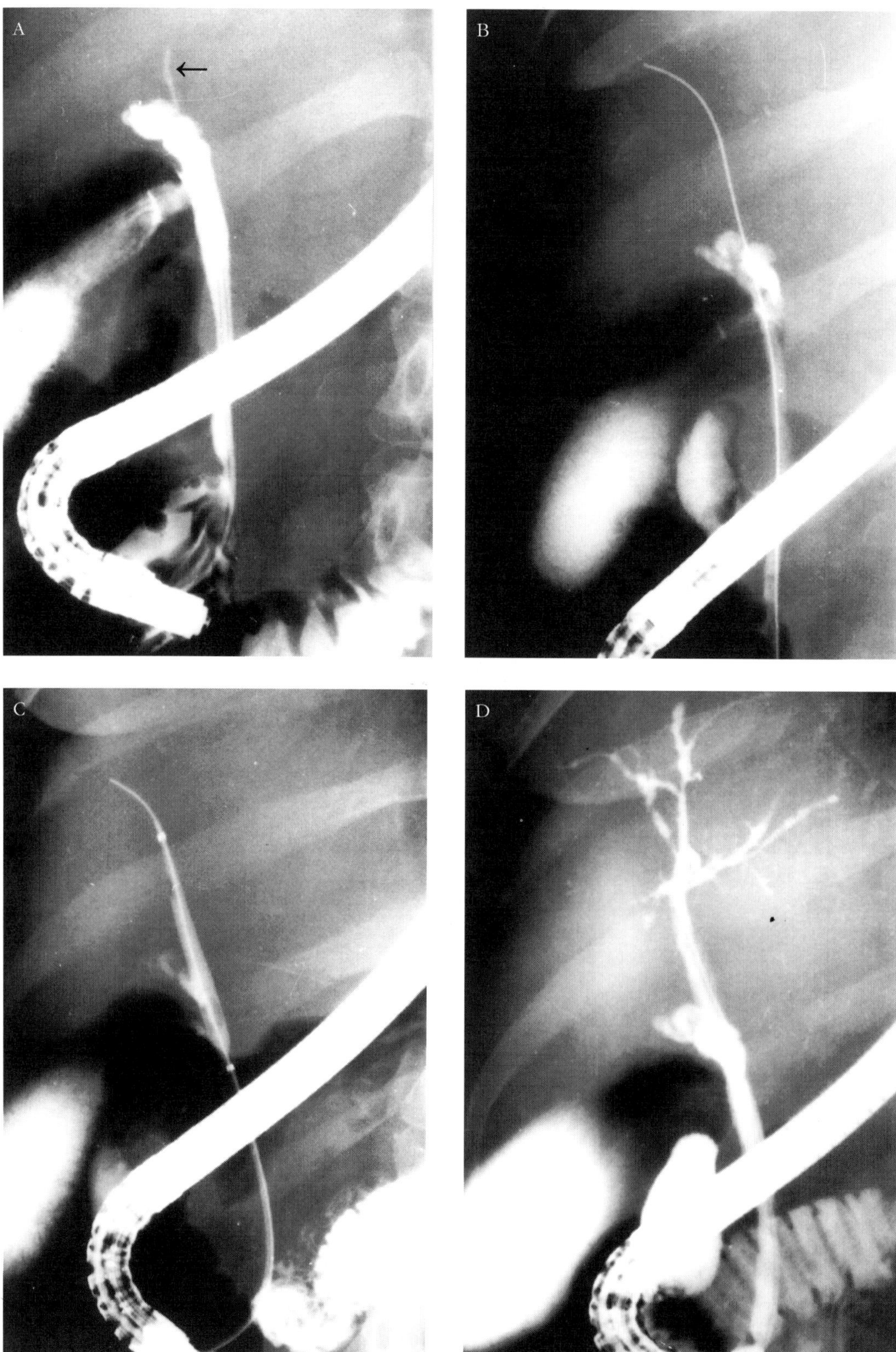

**_Figure 3.5_**
Sclerosing cholangitis in a 19-year-old male with ulcerative colitis. (A) Normal common bile duct. Severe narrowing of the common hepatic duct (↑) without visualization of the intrahepatic ducts. (B) A guide wire is introduced into the right hepatic duct. (C) The tapered balloon is fully inflated for 3 minutes. (D) Cholangiogram obtained immediately after dilation. The common hepatic duct now measures 5 mm in diameter. Irregular areas of stenosis and ectasia of the right intrahepatic ducts are visualized.

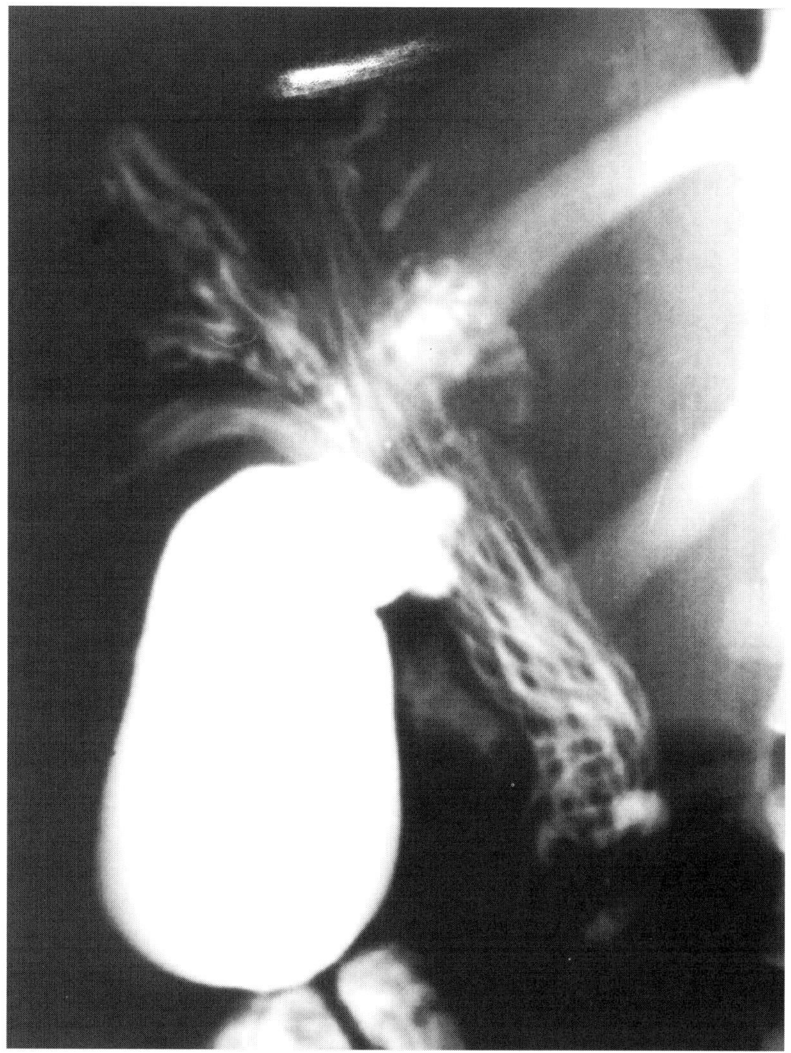

***Figure 3.6***
*Ascaris* in the common bile duct in a 17-year-old jaundiced female
with biliary colic. Multiple tubular filling defects are visualized in the
common duct and in the intrahepatic ducts.

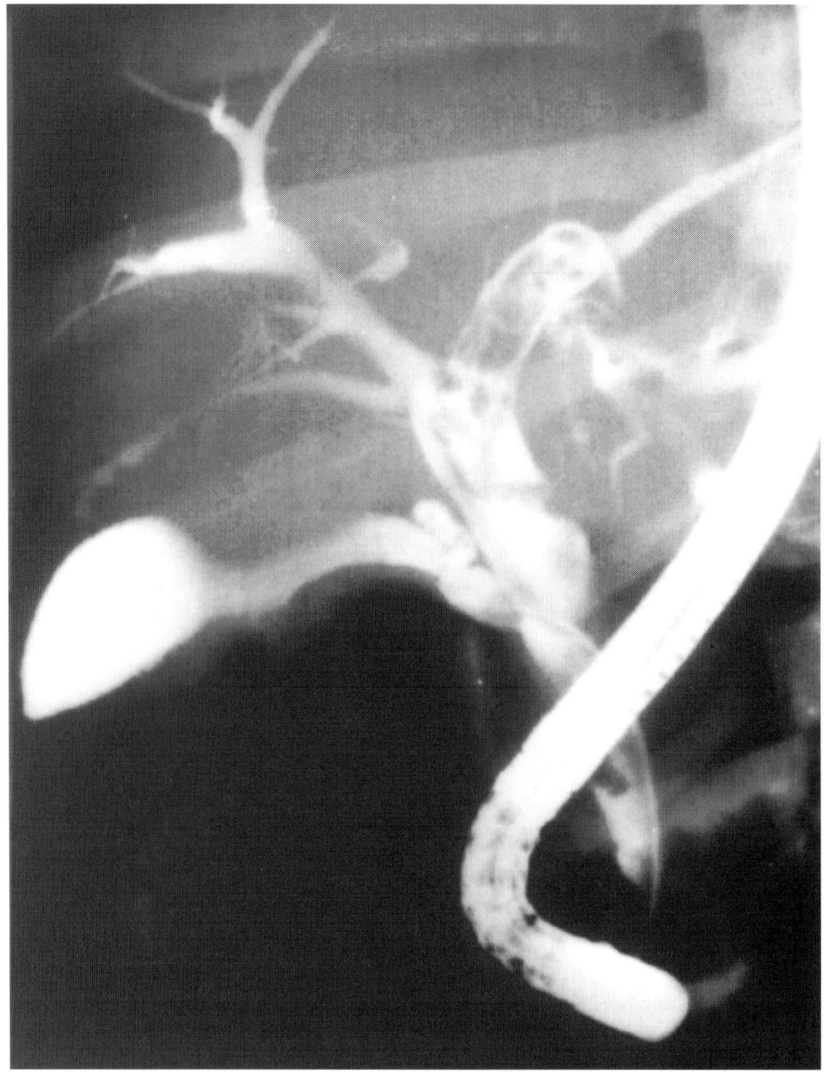

***Figure 3.7***
Dead *Ascaris* in the common bile duct. Multiple filling defects are visualized. After endoscopic sphincterotomy, multiple dead worms are extracted with a balloon.

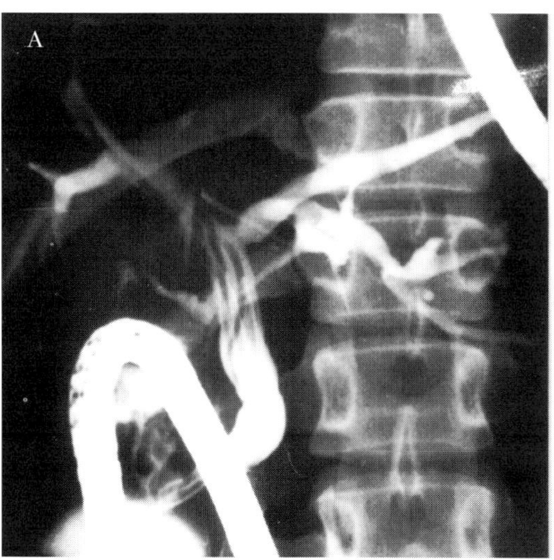
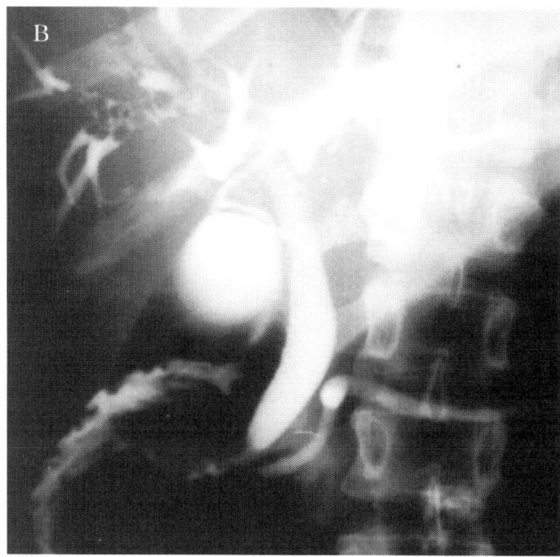

**Figure 3.8**

*Ascaris* in the common bile duct in a 18-year-old male with biliary colic and jaundice. (A) At least four tubular filling defects are visible in the common bile duct and one is located in the right hepatic duct. (B) Dilated common bile duct after endoscopic removal of worms.

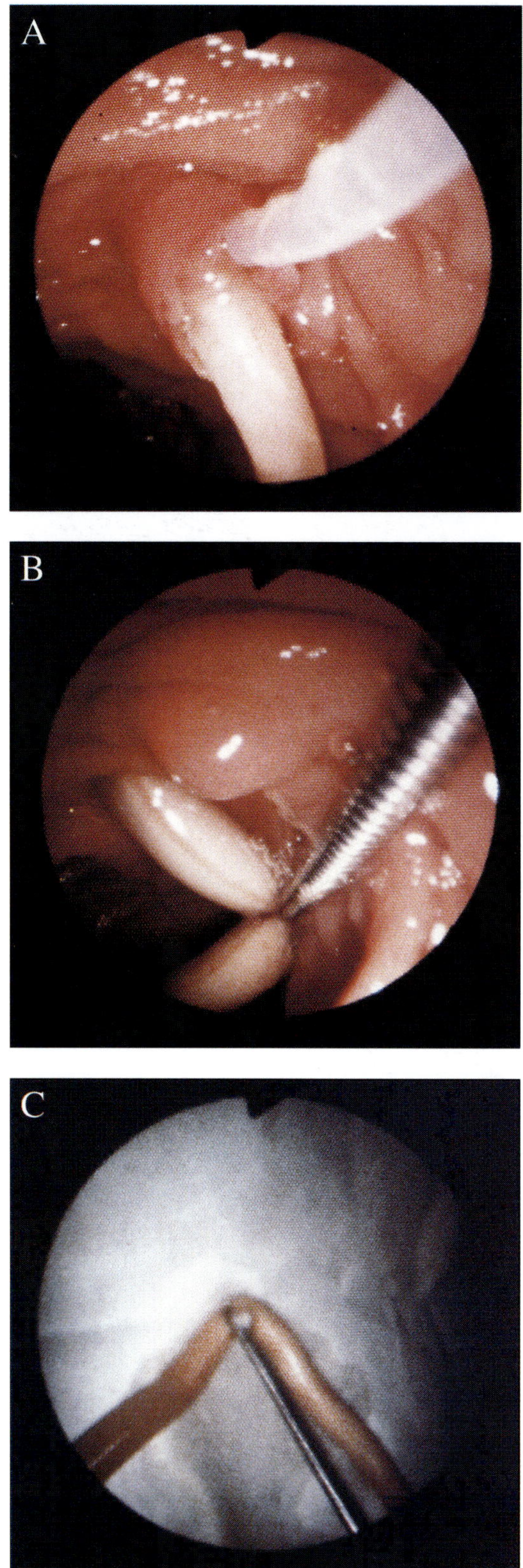

**Figure 3.9**
*Ascaris* in the common bile duct and endoscopic treatment. (A) Round worm protruding from the papillary orifice beside the cannula. (B) A tripod device captures the worm. (C) After retiring the endoscope, the *Ascaris* can be observed.

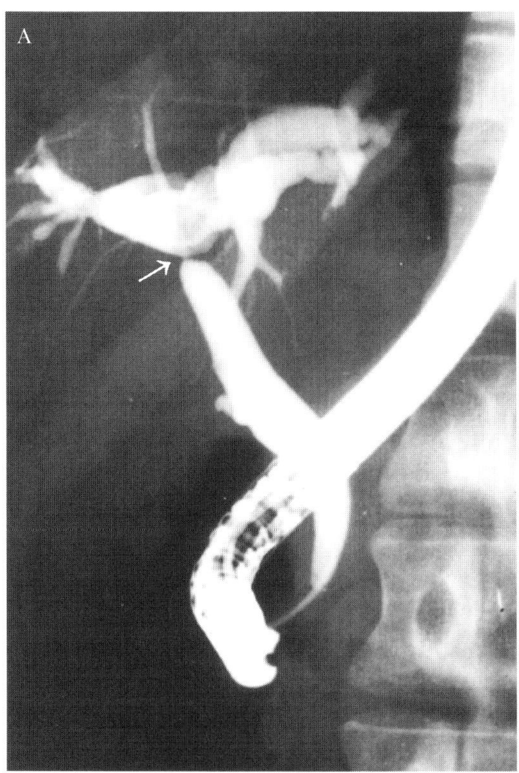

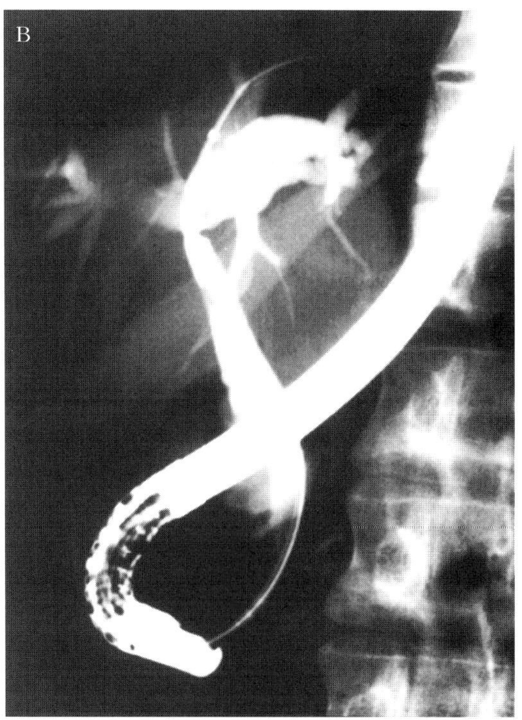

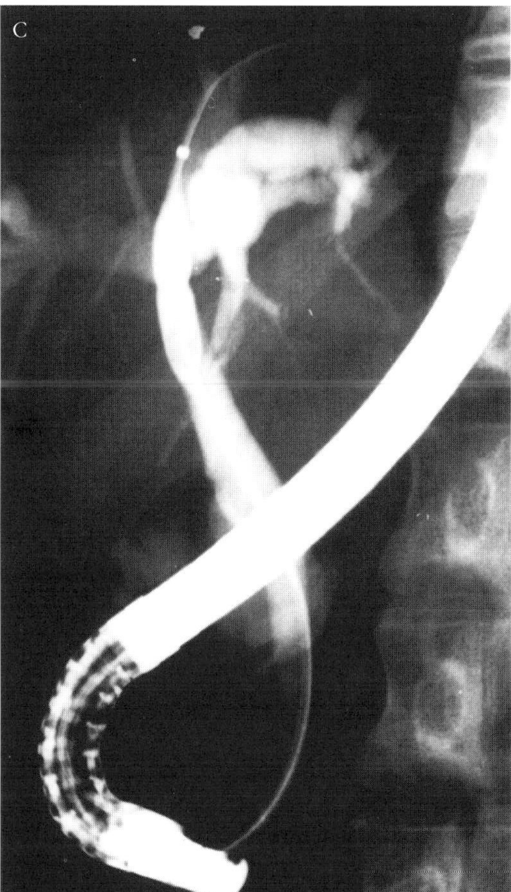

***Figure 3.10***

Benign common hepatic duct stricture. (A): Normal common bile duct. Filiform narrowing (↑) at the junction of both hepatic ducts with the common hepatic duct. Dilatation of the intrahepatic ducts. (B) Stricture dilation with a 6-French hydrostatic balloon. (C) Stricture dilation with a 8-French hydrostatic balloon.

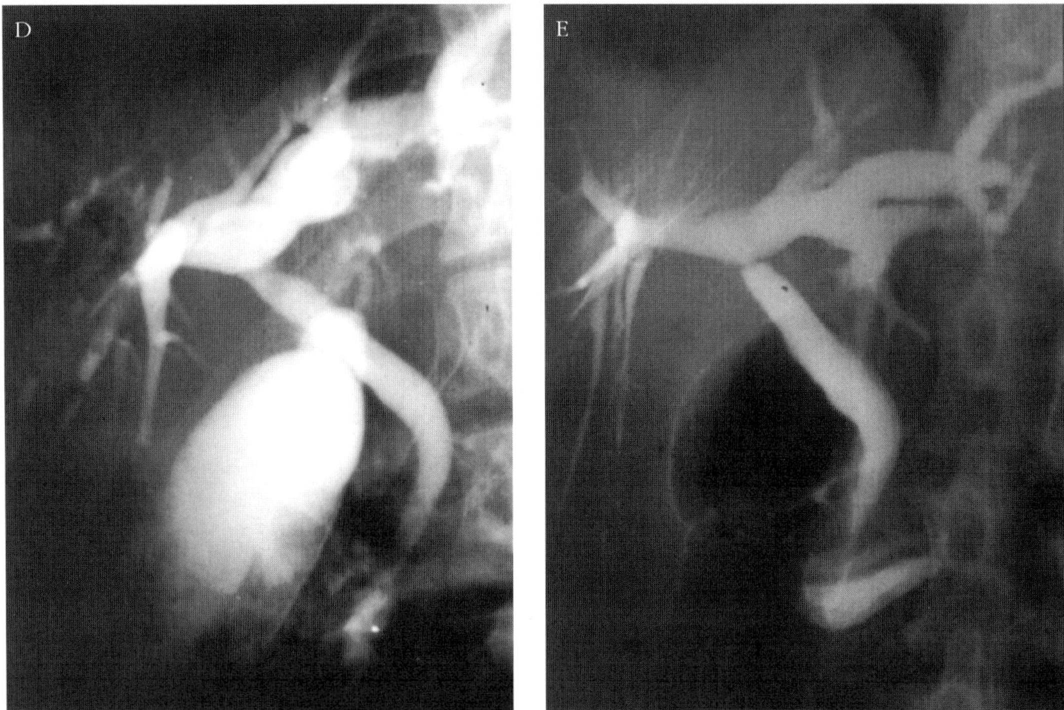

***Figure 3.10 (contd.)***
Benign common hepatic duct stricture. (D) After dilation, the stricture is wide open. (E)
After a follow-up period of 4 years the patient developed another attack of acute cholangitis.
A repeated ERCP demonstrated dilated intrahepatic ducts and a persistent wide web.
Surgical excision of this web was curative.

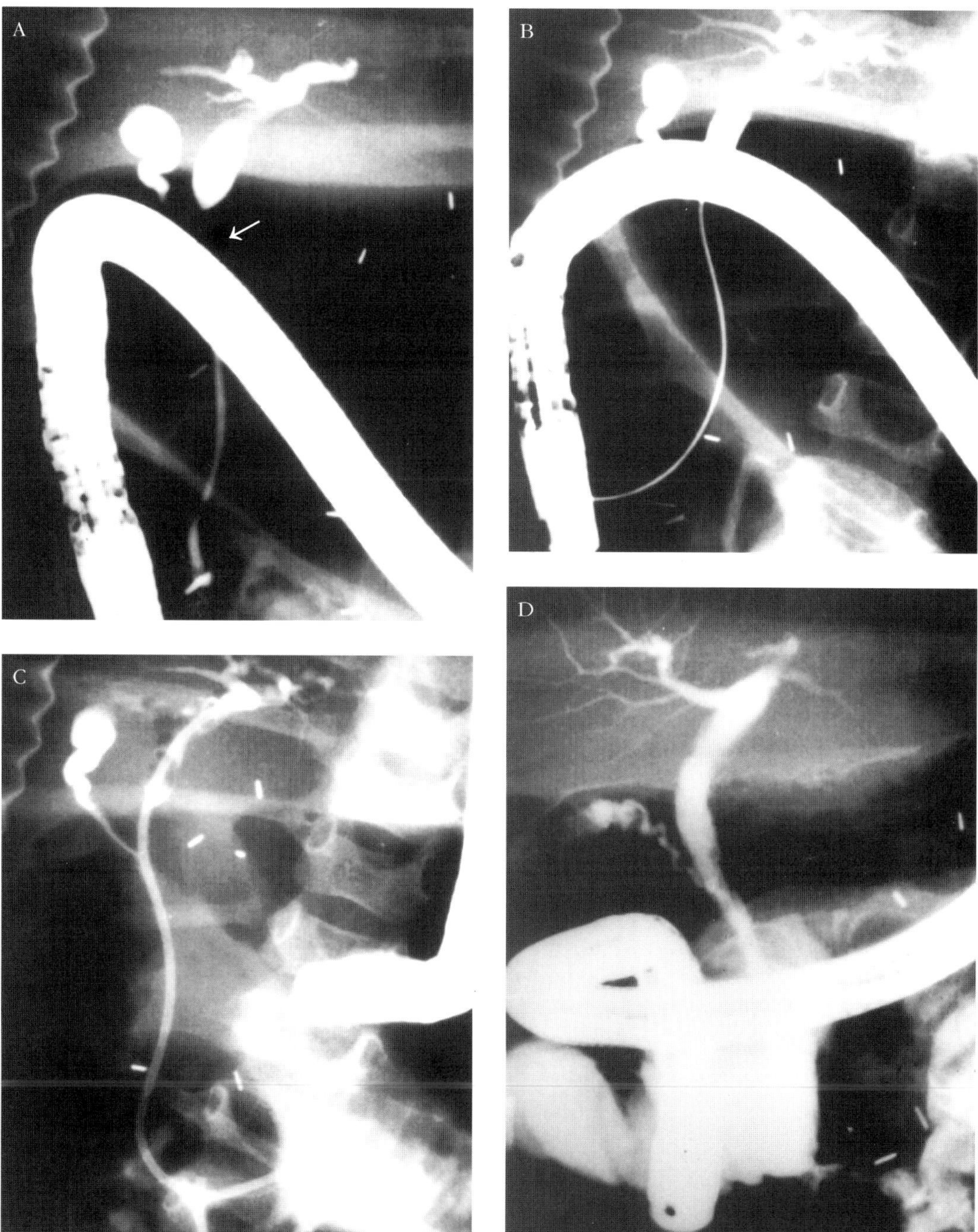

***Figure 3.11***

Malignant stricture at the common hepatic duct in a 21-month-old male due to an adrenal neuroblastoma. (A) Stricture at the common hepatic duct (↑) with dilatation of intrahepatic ducts. Normal common bile duct. (B) A guide wire is introduced into the left hepatic duct. (C) A 7-French double-pigtail biliary stent is placed. (D) After 4 months with chemotherapy, the biliary stent was removed and the common hepatic duct looked slightly dilated without stricture.

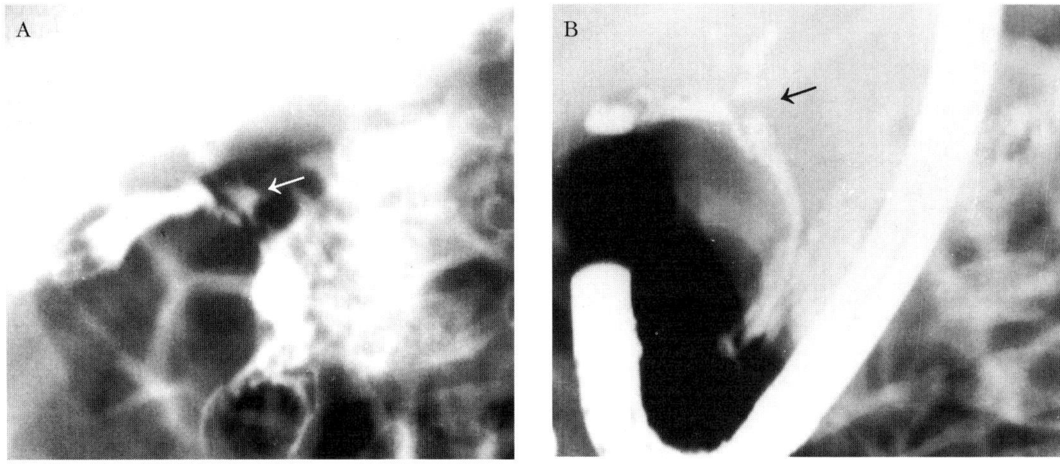

***Figure 3.12***
Choledocholithiasis. (A) Choledocholithiasis in a 62-day-old jaundiced infant with hemolytic anemia. Common bile duct stone (↑) with a dilated common duct and multiple gallbladder stones. (B) Choledocholithiasis in a 29-day-old neonate with hemolytic anemia. Common bile duct stone (↑) with intrahepatic ducts dilatation.

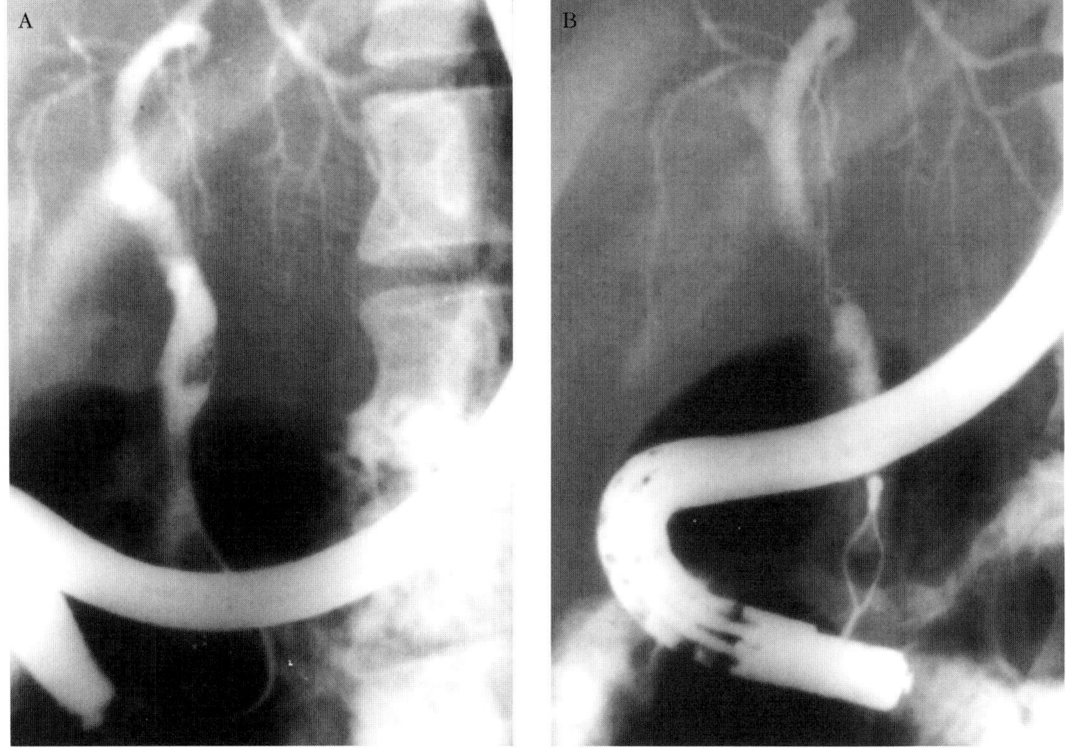

***Figure 3.13***
Choledocholithiasis and endoscopic stone removal in a 12-year-old female with previous cholecystectomy. (A) Common bile duct stone. (B) After endoscopic sphincterotomy, a basket is introduced into the common duct to extract the stone.

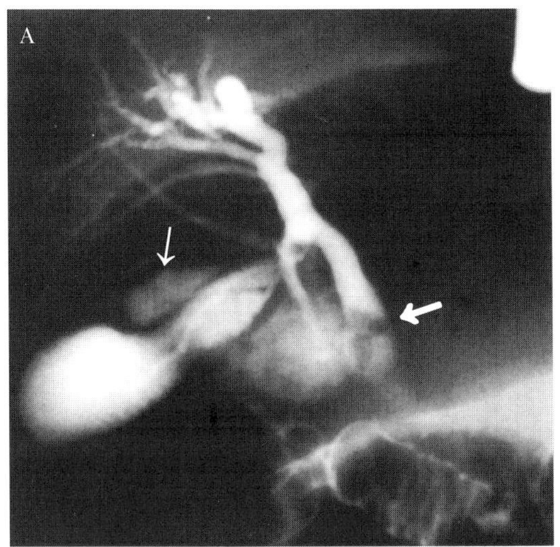
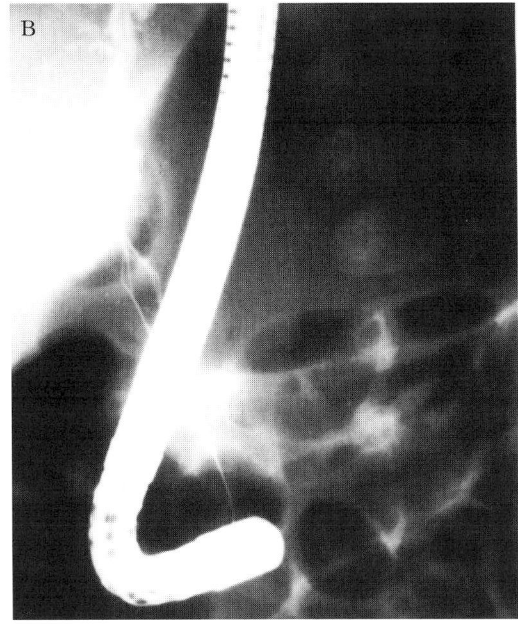

**_Figure 3.14_**

Choledocholithiasis and endoscopic stone removal in a 6-month-old jaundiced infant with sepsis. (A) Large filling defect (↑) within a dilated common bile duct. Two gallbladders (↑) arising from the same cystic duct. Intrahepatic ducts dilation. (B) After endoscopic sphincterotomy a basket is introduced into the common bile duct to remove the stone.

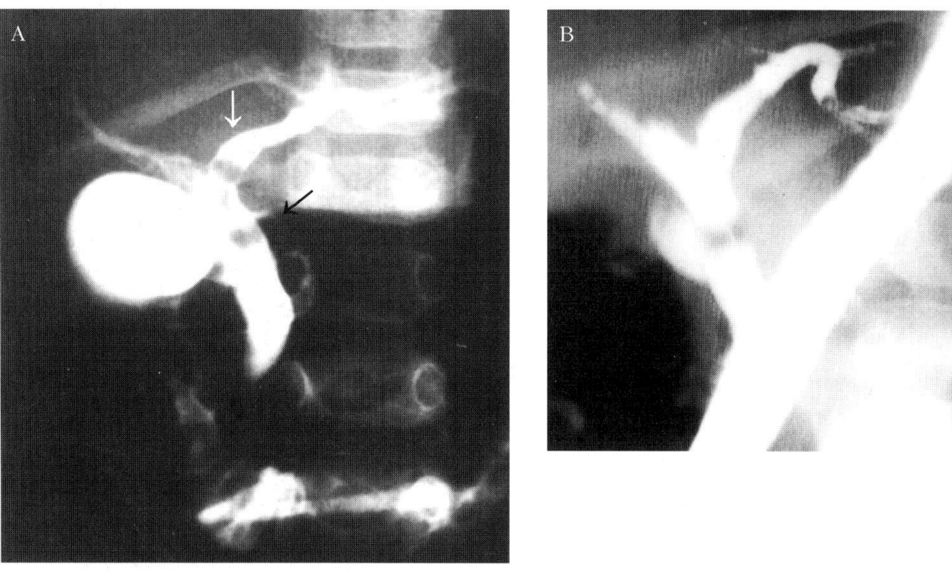

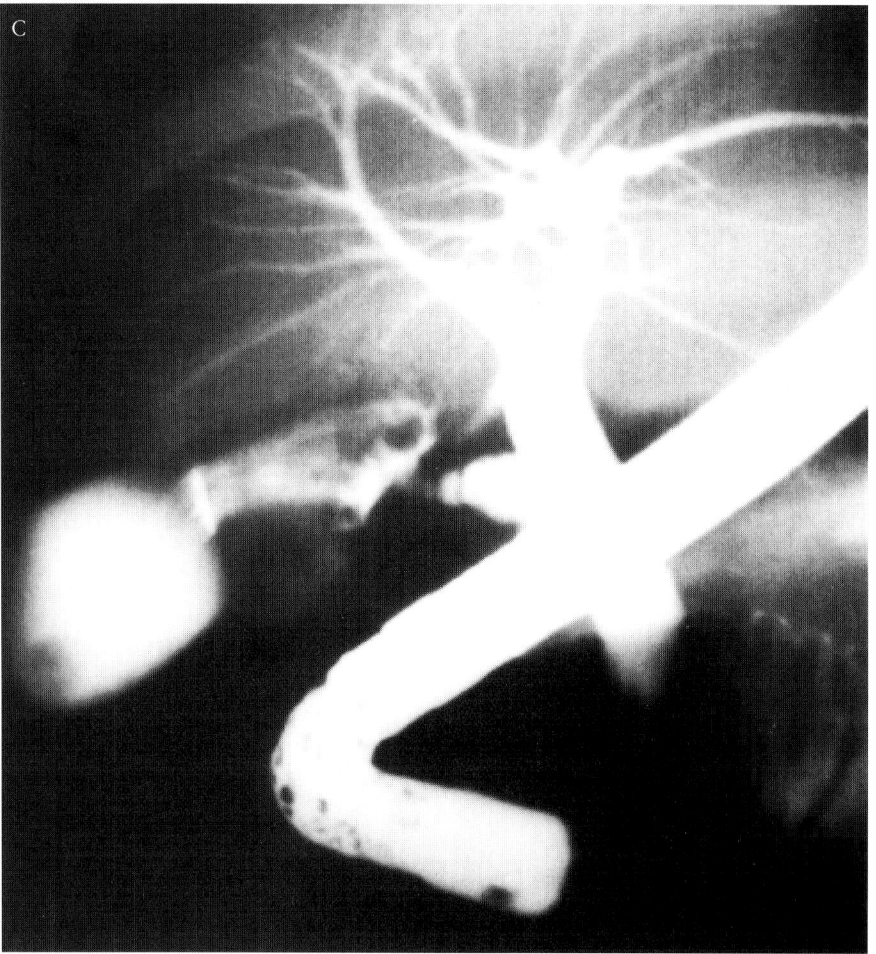

***Figure 3.15***

Choledocholithiasis in a 9-month-old infant treated by combined endoscopic sphincterotomy and laparoscopic cholecystectomy. (A) Multiple common bile duct stones (↑) within a dilated common duct and intrahepatic ducts. (B) After endoscopic sphincterotomy a balloon is introduced into the common duct to remove the stones. (C) After removing the common duct stones no filling defects are seen. The gallbladder is visualized with multiple stones. A laparoscopic cholecystectomy was performed at age 21 months.

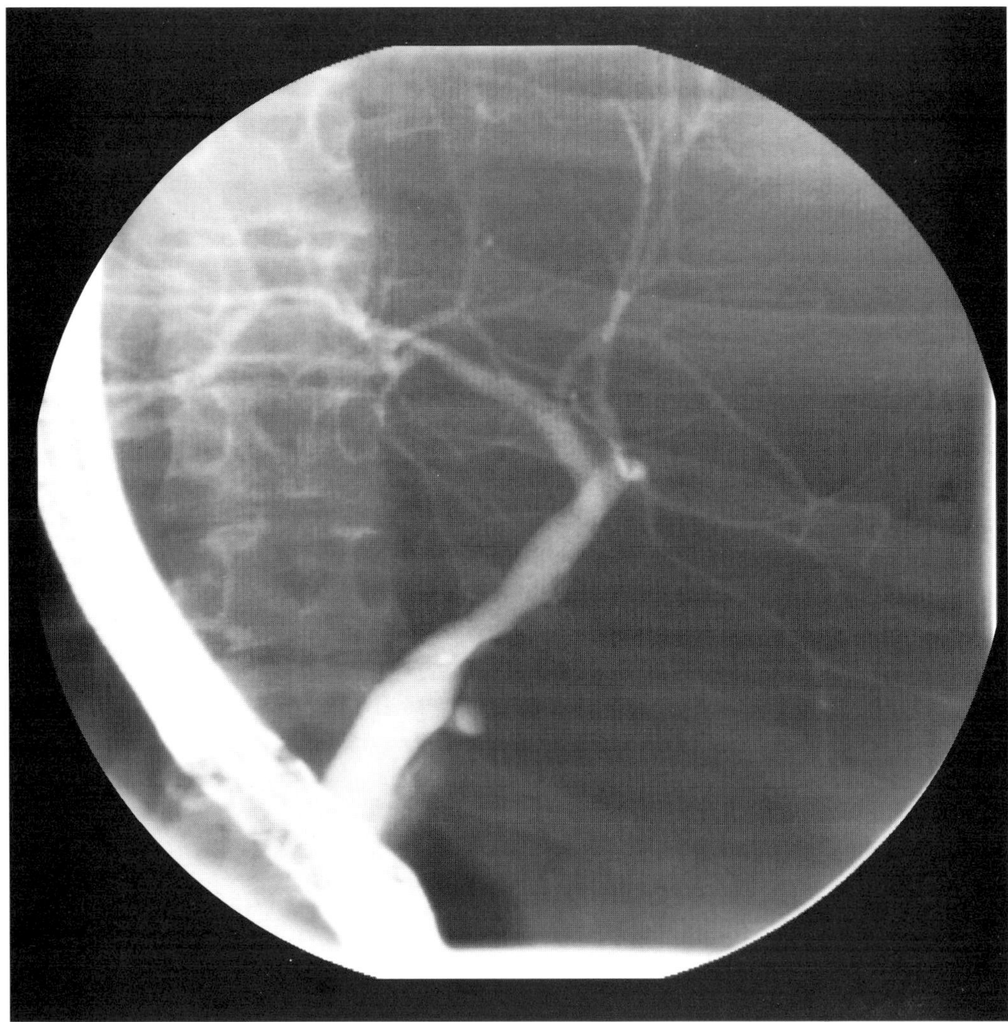

***Figure 3.16***
Cholangiogram in an 18-year-old female with progressive jaundice after liver transplantation. Some degree of bile duct caliber change, although no stricture, is seen in the region of the duct to duct anastomosis. Note the two ligated cystic duct remnants on donor and recipient portions of the bile duct.

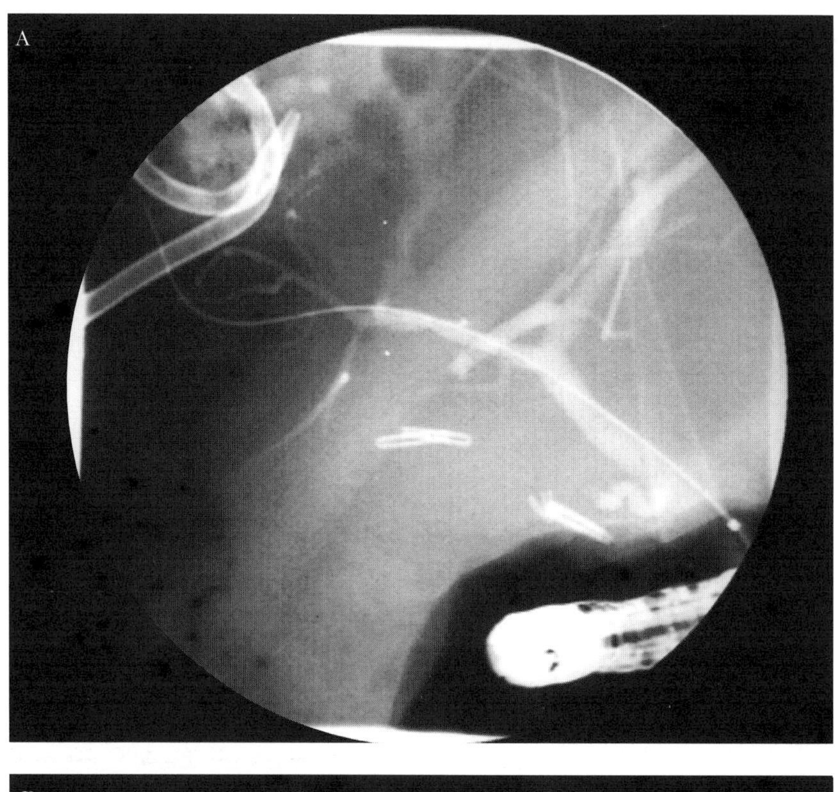

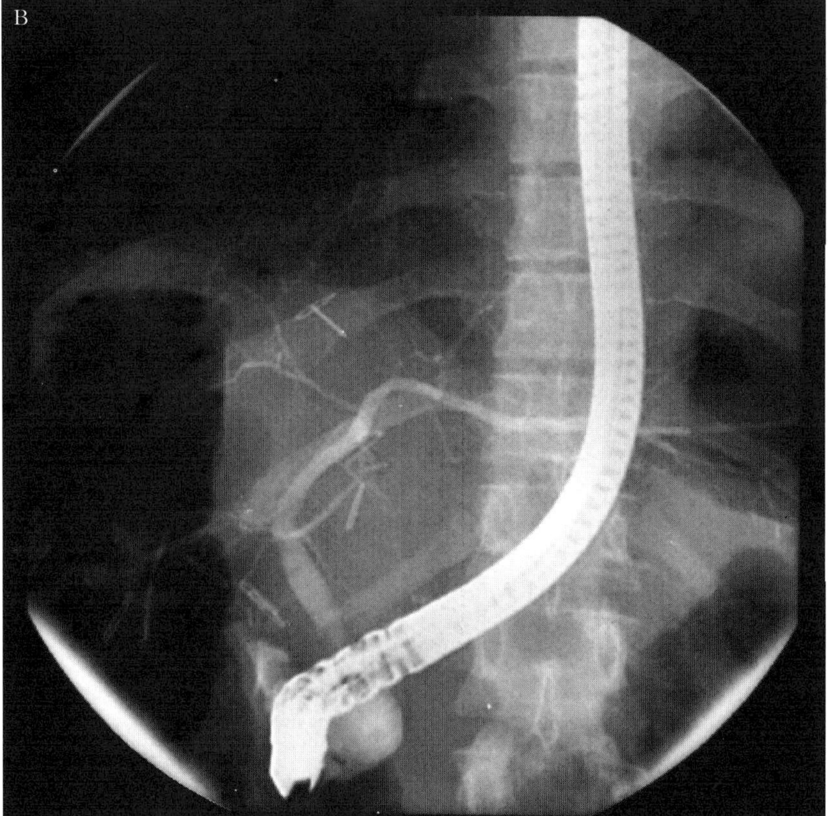

**Figure 3.17**

Cholangiogram in an 18-year-old male with residual intrahepatic bile leak after abdominal trauma. (A) Contrast extravasating from a branch of the right hepatic duct. Note the guidewire passing through the site of duct disruption, and the pigtail catheter draining fluid collection. A short transpapillary stent (2 cm long, 10 French) was placed. (B) Repeat cholangiogram 3 months later shows resolution of bile leak (courtesy of Dr. P Moses).

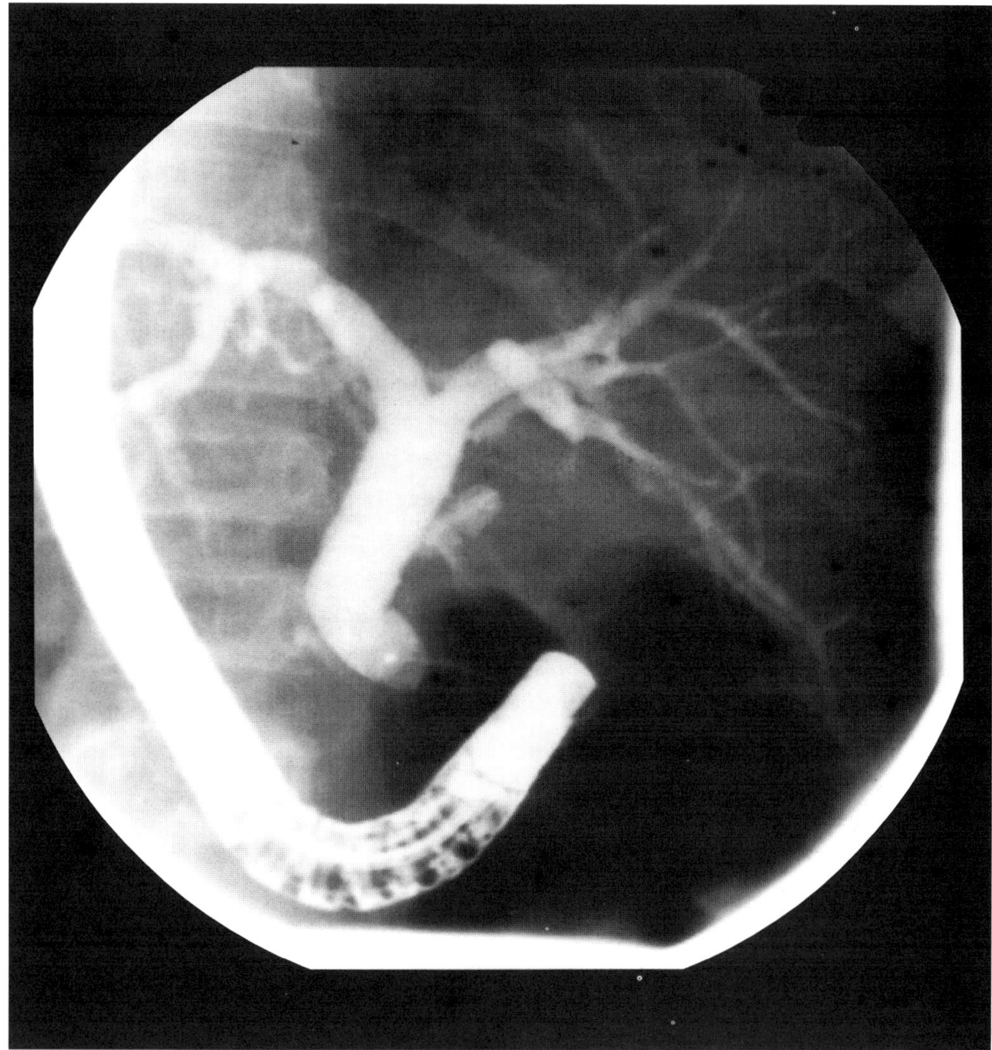

***Figure 3.18***
Dilated bile duct secondary to papillary stenosis in a 13-year-old male with AIDS and Cryptosporidium-positive stools.

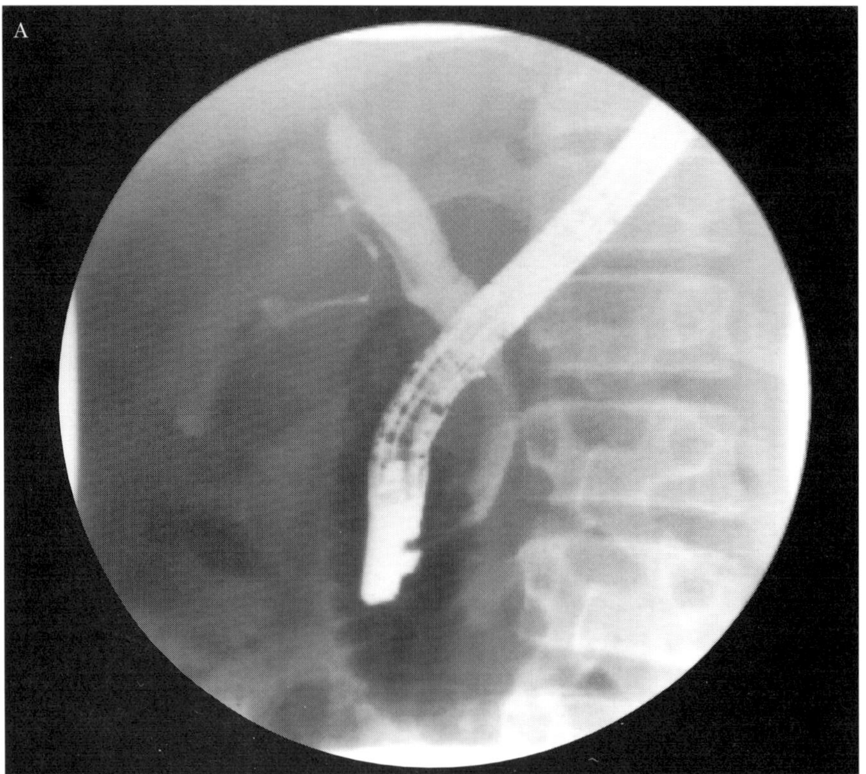

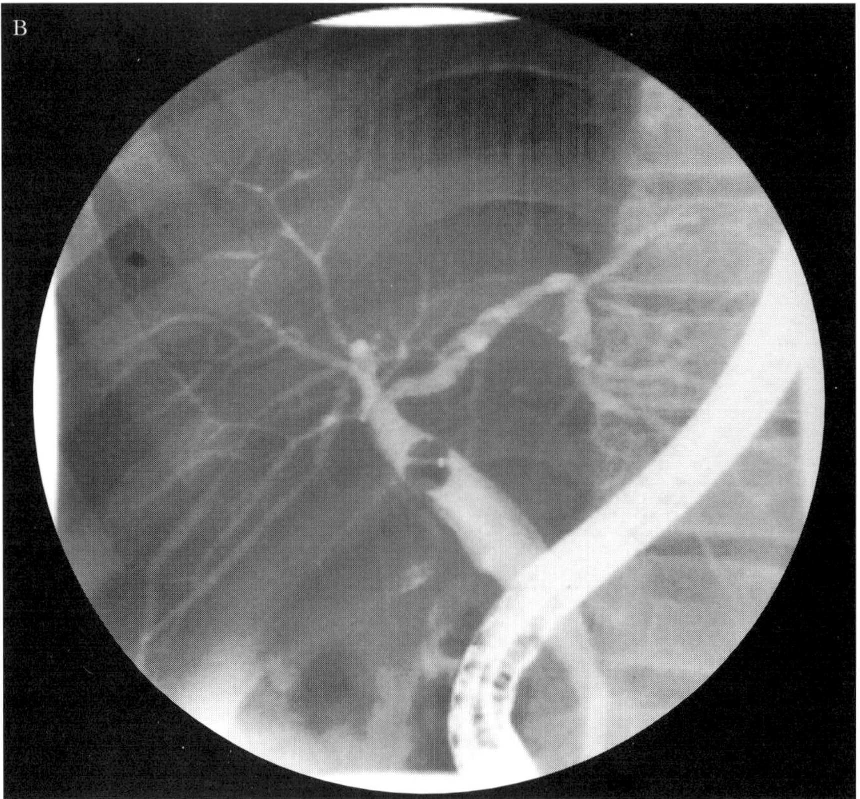

### *Figure 3.19*

Cholangiogram in 13-year-old male with Crohn's disease and sclerosing cholangitis. (A) Initial contrast injection during deep bile duct cannulation shows dilated extrahepatic ducts but no filling of intrahepatic ducts. (B) Repeat injection with retrieval balloon catheter allows filling of intrahepatic ducts demonstrating diffuse ductal irregularities.

# PART II

# ERCP in diseases of the pancreas

# CHAPTER 4

# Recurrent pancreatitis (obstructive causes)

Recognition of recurrent pancreatitis is often delayed in children because of a low index of clinical suspicion for this entity. The disease is characterized by episodes of acute pancreatitis, manifested by unexplained recurrent abdominal pain followed by asymptomatic intervals of varying duration. Diagnosis may be missed for several months or years. Patients are treated supportively during the acute attack and, if no exact cause is found, discharged without specific treatment. Two general categories of recurrent pancreatitis have been described: (i) non-obstructive: hereditary (Alpha 1-antitrypsin deficiency, aminoaciduria, hyperparathyroidism, hemochromatosis), cystic fibrosis, hyperlipidemia (types I and V), medication, eosinophilic pancreatitis, collagen-vascular diseases and Crohn's disease (1–6), and (ii) obstructive causes (7–16). If no specific cause is identified, such cases may be classified as idiopathic recurrent pancreatitis.

New insights into the ductal system through ERCP have increasingly directed our attention to morphologic changes of the pancreatic duct. ERCP offers the definition of the common bile duct and pancreatic ductal system that is necessary to make the decisions in the management of children with recurrent pancreatitis. Whatever the etiology of pancreatitis, the possibility of an anatomic abnormality amenable to endoscopic therapy or surgery should always be considered (17). ERCP has been found useful in the identification of treatable causes in 40% of adults (18) and in 45% to 95% of children with idiopathic recurrent pancreatitis (19–25) (Table 4.1). Unlike pancreatitis in adults, there were no causes of alcoholic pancreatitis and few idiopathic cases. It needs to be emphasized that pancreatitis in children is often a surgically (26) or endoscopically correctable disease (25).

**Table 4.1** Frequency of treatable causes in ERCP in children and adolescents with recurrent pancreatitis

| Author, year (reference) | No. of patients | Treatable causes in ERCP |
| --- | --- | --- |
| Forbes, 1984 (19) | 25 | 21 (84%) |
| Buckley, 1990 (20) | 18 | 8 (45%) |
| Putnam, 1991 (21) | 12 | 9 (75%) |
| Dite, 1992 (22) | 16 | 13 (81%) |
| Brown, 1994 (23) | 9 | 7 (75%) |
| Lemmel, 1994 (24) | 29 | 28 (95%) |
| Guelrud, 1994 (25) | 50 | 37 (74%) |
| Total | 159 | 123 (77%) |

# Congenital disorders

## Biliary anomalies

### Choledochal cyst

Choledochal cysts have been associated with recurrent pancreatitis (27,28). Proposed mechanisms of pancreatitis include (i) pancreatic duct obstruction by the cyst, (ii) reflux of bile into the pancreatic duct, and (iii) increased pancreatic ductal pressure due to sphincter of Oddi dysfunction. ERCP has found an association of choledochal cyst and recurrent pancreatitis in approximately 10% of children evaluated by ERCP (19–25) (Table 4.2). Shirai *et al.* (29) performed ERCP in six infants with choledochal cyst and abnormal pancreaticobiliary junction and four had recurrent pancreatitis. We have found severe pancreatic duct abnormalities in patients with choledochal cysts associated with recurrent pancreatitis (Figs 4.1–4.4). Two patients had coexistence of choledochal cyst and pancreas divisum (Fig. 4.5).

**Table 4.2** Frequency of choledochal cyst in children with recurrent pancreatitis

| Author, year (reference) | No. of patients | No. of choledochal cysts |
|---|---|---|
| Forbes, 1984 (19) | 25 | 2 (8%) |
| Buckley, 1990 (20) | 18 | 1 (6%) |
| Putnam, 1991 (21) | 25 | 2 (8%) |
| Dite, 1992 (22) | 22 | 1 (6%) |
| Brown, 1994 (23) | 9 | 1 (11%) |
| Lemmel, 1994 (24) | 29 | 0 |
| Guelrud, 1994 (25) | 50 | 9 (18%) |
| Total | 159 | 17 (11%) |

Type III choledochal cyst or choledochocele (Fig. 4.6) has been reported in patients with recurrent pancreatitis (30). The youngest reported case was a 3-year-old female with chronic pancreatitis (31). The cause of recurrent pancreatitis associated with choledochocele is unclear. In some patients the cause of pancreatitis seemed to be increased pancreatic ductal pressure due to sphincter of Oddi dysfunction (32,33) similar to the motor abnormalities found in papillary stenosis (34) and in idiopathic recurrent pancreatitis (35).

As in patients with biliary symptoms and choledochal cysts, endoscopic treatment is probably not indicated. In selected cases, with fusiform choledochal cyst and a widely dilated common channel, endoscopic sphincterotomy with or without stone extraction can be safely performed with excellent results (25) (Figs 4.7 and 4.8).

Management of children with symptomatic choledochocele and recurrent pancreatitis is controversial. The goal of therapy is to establish effective drainage of the pancreatic duct. This objective can be achieved by endoscopic sphincterotomy (32,36) or operative laparotomy (30,37). We have treated one child with recurrent pancreatitis and choledochocele by endoscopic sphincterotomy with excellent results after a follow-up of 3 years (25).

### Anomalous pancreaticobiliary union

Anomalous union of the pancreaticobiliary ductal system has been associated with recurrent pancreatitis (Fig. 4.9) (37, 38). Gibson *et al.* (39) described a 3-year-old girl who had a choledochal cyst with pancreatitis found at operation. Reffensperger *et al.* (40) found similar findings in two girls and suggested that the reflux of bile into the pancreatic duct was the most likely cause of pancreatitis. Suda *et al.* (41) reported the histologic findings of the pancreas in 21 cases of anomalous pancreaticobiliary junction and 63 cases of an experimental animal model. They concluded that regurgitation of bile into the pancreatic duct does not always produce pancreatitis. The most important factor producing pancreatic injury was the presence of infected bile or activation of pancreatic enzymes when the long common channel is obstructed by cholelithiasis, protein plug or sphincter of Oddi spasm. A pancreatic or biliary ductal abnormality was found in 16 of 35 patients with recurrent pancreatitis in a series of children and adults who underwent ERCP (42,43). Surgical approach was based on the ERCP findings of potentially correctable lesions in these patients. Guelrud *et al.* (25) described the usefulness of ERCP in 50 children and adolescents with recurrent pancreatitis. Abnormal pancreaticobiliary junction was found in 12 patients, nine patients had a coexistent choledochal cyst (Fig. 2.16, Chapter 2).

**Pancreatic anomalies**

*Normal pancreas variations*
In adults, the normal diameter of the main pancreatic duct is 4–5 mm in the head, decreasing to 3–4 mm in the body and 1–2 mm in the tail. In children, the normal diameter of the pancreatic duct varies with age (Fig. 4.10). In most cases, an accessory duct system located above the main duct can be visualized. The accessory duct drains the pancreatic secretion through the minor papilla, which is located cephalad to the major papilla. Frequently, one or more branches located inferior to the main duct drain the uncinate process. Normal variations of the pancreatic duct configuration are frequently observed (44) (Figs 4.11 to 4.16).

*Pancreas divisum*
Pancreas divisum is a congenital anomaly caused by failure of fusion of the dorsal and ventral endodermal buds during the sixth and seventh weeks of gestation. Each duct drains via its own separate orifice: the major papilla of Vater for the ventral duct of Wirsung and the minor accessory papilla for the dorsal duct of Santorini. The ventral pancreas becomes the inferior portion of the head of the pancreas. The dorsal gland forms the superior part of the head, as well as the body and tail. Normally the ductal systems fuse and the body and tail drain predominantly through the duct of Wirsung. The duct of Santorini recedes to a minor accessory role or even disappears entirely.

In some cases, a rudimentary, thin duct may communicate the ventral duct system with the dorsal pancreatic duct (45), resulting in incomplete pancreas divisum (Fig. 4.17). The incomplete pancreas divisum is encountered less often than pancreas divisum. It has been found in 1.2% of autopsy specimens (45) and in 0.13% (46), 0.9% (47), and 2% (48) in ERCP studies. The clinical significance of this anomaly is uncertain. As with pancreas divisum, this anatomic variant has been identified in healthy individuals and in patients with recurrent pancreatitis (Fig. 4.18–4.23). In incomplete pancreas divisum, visualization of the dorsal pancreatic duct is accomplished through a communicating branch of the ventral pancreas which may be insufficient to drain the pancreatic secretion of the dorsal pancreas during increased flow. If pancreatic changes are present, they usually involve the dorsal pancreatic duct (Fig. 4.24) and may cause pain and eventually recurrent pancreatitis. However, we have found isolated ventral chronic pancreatitis in incomplete pancreas divisum that cannot be explained by obstruction of the minor papilla (Fig. 4.25). In one patient, sphincter of Oddi dysfunction was demonstrated (Fig. 4.26) (49), suggesting an incomplete drainage of pancreatic secretion through the major papilla and may explain the chronic pancreatitis confined to the ventral pancreas. Recently, incomplete pancreas divisum was found in four children with idiopathic recurrent pancreatitis, suggesting a contributing etiologic role in pancreatitis. One child was treated by minor papilla sphincterotomy (50).

Pancreas divisum is the most common congenital anomaly of the pancreas. It has been found in 5–14% of autopsy series (51) and 0.3–8% of ERCP studies (52,53). In our experience with 272 consecutive cases of successful ERCP performed in children, pancreas divisum was found in nine (3.3%) children (54). Two patients' groups were identified on the basis of the age at which ERCP was performed. Group 1 included 147 neonates or young infants in which ERCP was performed to evaluate neonatal cholestasis. Two (1.4%) neonates had pancreas divisum, one with neonatal hepatitis (Fig. 4.27) and the other with biliary atresia (Fig. 4.28). Group 2 included 125 children older than 1 year and adolescents in which ERCP was performed to evaluate pancreatic and biliary disorders. Seven (5.6%) children had pancreas divisum. This anomaly was found more frequently in patients evaluated for recurrent pancreatitis (12%) than in patients evaluated for biliary disorders (1.3%).

The clinical significance of pancreas divisum is controversial since not all patients with this anomaly have clinical symptoms. Several authors (51,55–57) have suggested an association between pancreas divisum and pancreatitis, on the basis of inadequate drainage of the minor papilla. However, other authors have considered it to be a coincidental finding by reviewing large series of ERCP (58–60). Cotton showed a high incidence of the anomaly (25.6%) in patients with idiopathic pancreatitis, when compared with the incidence of 3.8% in "control" patients with biliary disease (61). In that study, the incidence in patients with gallstones may be falsely low, as not all endoscopists attempt to visualize the pancreatic ducts routinely in that context. Also, the incidence of pancreas divisum may appear high in a center if it attracts a selected population of patients with pancreatitis. Delhaye *et al.* reported their experience with 304 patients with pancreas divisum (60). They found no increased incidence of the anomaly among patients with pancreatitis. However, when they studied another group of 646 patients prospectively (61), there were 15 patients with pancreas divisum among 122 investigated for pancreatitis. This incidence of 12% is almost twice that found in patients with miscellaneous conditions in which pancreas divisum was found in 38 of 524 (7%). However, lack of uniformity of data made it unlikely that epidemiological analysis alone would provide definitive answers.

The combination of this anomaly with accessory papilla stenosis may lead to a functional obstruction. The finding of elevated pressure in the dorsal duct of some patients with pancreas divisum supports this hypothesis (52,62). However, it cannot estimate the functional adequacy of the accessory papilla. Warshaw *et al.* (63) measured the size of the accessory orifice by probing at surgery and proposed 0.75 mm as a lower limit of normal. Other surgeons have not reproduced this finding. The inability to cannulate the accessory papilla is not a useful criteria for obstruction. With the catheters and techniques now in use, the dorsal pancreas can be visualized in approximately 90% of patients (60,64) and the duct is generally of normal caliber. Delayed drainage of the dorsal duct after ERCP has been reported (65) but is exceptional. The fact that the dorsal pancreatic duct is not dilated in symptomatic patients has been used as a criteria against the obstructive nature of this anomaly. However, ERCP is performed on an unstimulated resting gland, conditions that allowed the duct to empty and contract. It is possible that the degree of obstruction is partial and it is only after eating that an abnormal dilation occurs. This idea is the basis of the provocation test. Warshaw *et al.* (66) have suggested the use of a secretin stimulation test using ultrasonography to monitor dorsal duct size. While early duct dilatation occurs normally, prolonged dilation for 15–30 minutes was felt to be indicative of outflow obstruction. This observation has been contested by others and not confirmed (67). The finding of a dilatation at the termination of the dorsal duct called "Santorinicele" supports the theory that outflow obstruction at the minor papilla may cause pancreatitis (68). Further support for the obstruction-to-flow hypothesis comes from the observation that histologic and ductal morphologic changes may be segmental, isolated to the dorsal pancreas (51,54,65,69,70). Finally, advocates of this hypothesis support their theory based on the benefits reported in some series for dorsal duct decompression obtained surgically (71–73) or endoscopically (50,52,53,73–77). Patients most likely to benefit were those with recurrent acute pancreatitis. Patients with chronic pancreatitis did poorly after this therapy.

These series dealt specifically with adult patients. Many authors have argued that if pancreas divisum causes pancreatitis, one might expect the disease to occur much earlier in life. Some reports (57,78) suggest that pancreatitis associated with pancreas divisum occurs earlier in life than other forms of pancreatitis. This has been denied by others (60). In children with recurrent pancreatitis, pancreas divisum has been found in 10% of patients (Table 4.3).

**Table 4.3** Frequency of pancreas divisum in children with recurrent pancreatitis

| Author, year (reference) | No. of patients | No. of patients with pancreas divisum |
|---|---|---|
| Forbes, 1984 (19) | 25 | 4 (16%) |
| Buckley, 1990 (20) | 18 | 1 (5%) |
| Putnam, 1991 (21) | 12 | 0 |
| Dite, 1992 (22) | 16 | 1 (6%) |
| Brown, 1994 (23) | 9 | 2 (22%) |
| Lemmel, 1994 (24) | 29 | 2 (7%) |
| Guelrud, 1994 (25) | 50 | 6 (12%) |
| Total | 159 | 16 (10%) |

ERCP is mandatory in the diagnosis of pancreas divisum. Cannulation of the main papilla shows a short duct of Wirsung (ventral pancreas) that quickly tapers and undergoes arborization (Fig. 4.29). To confirm the diagnosis it is most important to cannulate the accessory papilla to demonstrate the dorsal pancreas. Cannulation of the accessory papilla must be carried out very carefully. The target orifice is usually of pinpoint size. The use of a needle-tipped catheter (23-gauge needle, e.g. Cremer catheter) has proved superior to the standard fine-tipped polyethylene catheters (19,79,80). Cannulation of the accessory papilla with dorsal pancreas ductography is successfully accomplished in approximately 80% of attempts when the needle-tipped catheter is used (79). Blind probing with the needle catheter traumatizes the tiny papilla and makes recognition of the papilla orifice more difficult. Cannulation is best achieved from a long endoscopic position as it permits more perpendicular viewing of the accessory papilla from a close distance. Cannulation is achieved by impacting the needle tip within the papilla without deeper penetration. A potential complication from this catheter equipped with a short needle is submucosal injection of contrast media that could result in pancreatitis. Submucosal injection occurred in 19% of pancreas divisum patients without clinical sequelae (79). While the needle catheter greatly facilitates cannulation of the accessory papilla, a more basic obstacle to cannulation of the orifice is often encountered in trying to locate it. The use of intravenous secretin which stimulates pancreatic secretion through the accessory papilla has been proposed. In 15 patients with divisum, the accessory papilla was not visible in four cases until the administration of secretion stimulated a brisk outpouring of fluid from an otherwise non-apparent opening (64). Pancreatic duct abnormalities may be present in patients with divisum and pancreatitis. If changes are present, they usually involve only the dorsal pancreatic duct. This may sometimes result in narrowing of the distal common bile duct (Fig. 4.25). Pancreatic pseudocysts can occasionally be seen in the dorsal pancreas (Fig. 4.30).

Interventional treatment in patients with pancreas divisum is applied to patients whose symptoms are disabling. The treatment of symptomatic pancreas divisum was initially a surgical approach. Warshaw *et al.* performed minor papilla sphincteroplasty in 88 patients with symptomatic pancreas divisum and recurrent pancreatitis (71). Overall, 70% improved at a mean follow-up of 53 months. Yedlin *et al.* described a 10-year-old boy with pancreas divisum and recurrent pancreatitis for whom surgical intervention was successful (10). Wagner and Golladay performed double sphincteroplasties of minor and major sphincters in three children with recurrent pancreatitis with good results in a follow-up period of 12 months to 4 years (8). Adzick *et al.* performed minor papilla sphincteroplasty and cholecystectomy in four children with pancreas divisum and recurrent pancreatitis. All patients remained asymptomatic over the first post-operative year (81). Warshaw *et al.* treated two adolescents with pancreas divisum and recurrent acute pancreatitis by papillotomy of the minor papilla. They remained asymptomatic during follow-up of 19 and 67 months (63). One 9-year-old child with pancreas divisum and chronic pancreatitis had a Puestow operation with good results for a period of 20 months.

More recently, endoscopic treatment has been utilized to decompress the dorsal duct by a variety of methods: hydrostatic balloon dilation of the minor papilla (82), insertion of endoprostheses and sphincterotomy of the minor papilla with or without insertion of endoprosthesis. McCarthy *et al.* treated 19 patients with pancreas divisum using dorsal pancreatic stents and obtained 89% of improvement (83). Lans *et al.* reported the results of a randomized control trial of long-term (12 months) stenting of the minor papilla in patients with recurrent pancreatitis (84). Stents were changed every 4 months. Follow-up continued for at least 12 months after stent removal. Patients with stents had fewer episodes of pancreatitis and were more frequently judged to be improved (90% vs 11% of controls, $P < 0.05$). A temporary trial of stenting the dorsal duct has been used to decide whether surgery is appropriate. Patients who improve after stenting may be candidates for more sustained relief with surgical decompression (74). Similar to surgical sphincteroplasty, minor papilla sphincterotomy has been used to treat pancreas divisum (75). Soehendra *et al.* treated six patients using a precut or needle-knife sphincterotome over a stent, obtaining 83% symptomatic improvement (76). Liguory *et al.* performed minor papilla sphincterotomy with ($n = 2$) and without ($n = 8$) dorsal pancreatic duct stenting in 10 patients with pancreatitis (54). Seven patients (70%) remained symptom-free during a 3- to 30-month follow-up period. Lehman *et al.* treated 52 patients with pancreas divisum by minor papilla sphincterotomy performed with a needle-knife over a previously placed dorsal pancreatic duct stent (77). Patients with recurrent acute pancreatitis benefited more frequently than those with chronic pancreatitis (76% vs 27%, $P = 0.01$). In contrast, Coleman *et al.* found that patients with chronic pancreatitis also had a significant benefit (60%, $P < 0.0001$) from minor papilla sphincterotomy and dorsal pancreatic stent placement (85). Patients with pancreatic type pain without pancreatic enzyme elevation do not improve after endoscopic treatment (77,85). Pancreatitis as a complication of therapy occurred between 13% and 43% of the procedures but was mild and could be managed conservatively.

Endoscopic treatment in children with pancreas divisum is scarcely reported. Lemmel *et al.* performed endoscopic sphincterotomy of the minor papilla with stent placement in the

Santorini duct in two children with recurrent pancreatitis and pancreas divisum and in two children with pancreaticobiliary pain with good results in three children (24). Guelrud *et al.* treated three children with pancreas divisum and recurrent pancreatitis with minor papilla sphincterotomy without stent placement (Fig. 4.31) and obtained excellent results in two during a 1 year follow-up period (25). In one adolescent with pancreas divisum and a communicating cyst with the dorsal pancreas, pancreatic drainage was performed by pancreatic sphincterotomy and a stent placement until the cyst resolved (Fig. 4.32). Recently, we treated two adolescents with pancreas divisum and recurrent pancreatitis with normal pancreatic duct by minor papilla sphincterotomy and placement of a pancreatic stent (Fig. 4.33), which was removed after 10 days. Both patients remained asymptomatic for the following 10 months. Fox *et al.* treated two patients with incomplete pancreas divisum with minor papilla sphincterotomy and temporary pancreatic stent (50). One patient improved and one required Puestow.

Many endoscopists are concerned about pancreatic ductal changes seen with the long-term use of plastic stents and the risk of stent-damage to the gland (Fig. 4.34) (86–88). Consequently, there has been a trend toward sphincterotomy without stent placement or with only brief stenting. Long-term results are lacking for this technique.

Overall, these results indicate that in certain patients with recurrent pain or pancreatitis and pancreas divisum, endoscopic therapy or surgical intervention can offer relief or improvement in symptoms.

*Annular pancreas*

Annular pancreas is a congenital anomaly in which a band of pancreatic tissue encircles the second portion of the duodenum. This congenital anomaly has an incidence of approximately 1 in 20,000 (89). The ERCP appearance of this anomaly has been reported in a series of four patients from Japan (90). The annular pancreas originates from the ventral pancreas. It is thought to arise from either the failure of a portion of the ventral pancreas to rotate during embryogenic development or from persistence of the left branch of the ventral ductal system. It is associated with duodenal obstruction. The relationship with pancreatitis is unclear. In 14 cases of annular pancreas reported in the English literature there were five cases with coexistent pancreas divisum suggesting that pancreas divisum occurs more often in the presence of annular pancreas than in the general population (Fig. 4.35) (91). This association may explain pancreatitis in some patients.

The diagnosis of annular pancreas is suggested by the finding of an extrinsic, eccentric defect on the lateral margin of the second portion of the duodenum seen on an upper gastrointestinal barium study. Obstruction may be present and the proximal duodenum is dilated. ERCP may visualize the ventral duct encircling the duodenum (Fig. 4.36). We have seen one child with annular pancreas associated with choledochal cyst (Fig. 4.37). In another young infant with recurrent acute pancreatitis, an anomalous pancreaticobiliary junction was observed (Fig. 4.38). Prior to the development of ERCP the definitive diagnosis was made only at surgery.

*Short pancreas*

Agenesis of a pancreatic bud, also called short pancreas, is an exceptionally rare finding. Only about 20 cases of this anomaly have been reported in adults in the English literature (92–94). Pediatric cases, also quite rare, have been reported (Fig. 4.39) (25). It has been associated with polysplenia syndrome (95) and calcifying pancreatitis (96), and involves only the dorsal pancreatic duct. It must be differentiated from a pancreatic atrophy secondary to chronic pancreatitis. Computerized tomography confirms the diagnosis by revealing the absence of pancreatic tissue in the region of the body and tail of the pancreas. While recurrent pain attacks have been reported in some patients, the cause of the pain is unknown and has been presumed secondary to an autonomic neuropathy in those patients with diabetes (93). In other patients, the abdominal pain was due to pancreatitis (94). It has been suggested that this congenital abnormality may predispose to recurrent bouts of pancreatitis and abdominal pain, as has been suggested in patients with pancreas divisum (50). Awareness of the entity of short pancreas is important in the evaluation of a short pancreatic duct on the ERCP image. Cannulation of the accessory papilla should be done before ascribing a case of possible pancreatic atresia to agenesis of the dorsal pancreas.

*Pancreatocele*
This entity has not been reported previously. Guelrud reported a 14-year-old patient with recurrent pancreatitis and cystic dilatation at the end of the pancreatic duct (Fig. 4.40) (25). The patient refused any treatment and she developed another bout of acute pancreatitis 13 months after the ERCP was performed. The term pancreatocele is suggested by analogy with choledochocele, which is believed to result from a combination of obstruction and weakness of the distal duct wall, either of which may be congenital or acquired.

**Duodenal anomalies**

*Duodenal or gastric duplication*
Duplication cysts of the gastrointestinal tract are rare congenital anomalies which are most often present in children and young adults. The clinical presentation of duodenal duplication cysts is diverse. It may be asymptomatic for many years. When they do become symptomatic, they show a variety of clinical presentations: obstruction of the duodenum due to the presence of the cyst in the intestinal lumen, necrosis and bleeding of the adjacent intestine due to pressure upon the mesenteric blood vessels, hemorrhage from the duplication cyst itself, abdominal pain due to distention of the cyst mass or ulceration of ectopic gastric mucosa which can be observed in 15% of the cysts, or recurrent pancreatitis due to intermittent obstruction of the pancreatic duct (14,15,97,98).

The majority of duodenal duplication cysts occur on the mesenteric border in the second portion of the duodenum. Histologically, duodenal duplications are covered both inside and outside by duodenal mucosa with a distinct layer of smooth muscle between. Duplication cysts are filled with clear fluid, although cysts which communicate with the papilla may contain bile, pancreatic juice or even gallstones. ERCP has been shown to be useful in the diagnostic evaluation of this entity as well as for definitive treatment (14,98). If the cyst is bulging into the intestinal lumen, a wide cystoduodenostomy can be performed with excellent results. However, obstruction of the duodenum might prevent endoscopic cannulation of the papilla.

*Duodenal diverticulum*
In adults, duodenal diverticulum may be associated with pancreatitis (99,100) when the diverticulum is located in the area of the ampulla of Vater. Although the pathogenesis of pancreatitis in such patients is unclear, it is possible that the diverticulum may obstruct pancreatic drainage. In some patients, sphincter of Oddi dysfunction has been found (101,102) and endoscopic sphincterotomy may be beneficial to prevent further attacks (103,104). There are no reports in children.

# Acquired disorders

## Parasitic infestation
Pancreatitis complicating *Ascaris* infestation occurs uncommonly in children (11). Usually it

is due to migration of the worm in the bile duct, producing transient obstruction of the papilla of Vater with acute pancreatitis. The worm rarely migrates into the main pancreatic duct causing recurrent pancreatitis (105) and rarely causes necrotizing pancreatitis (106). ERCP is an excellent tool in the diagnosis and treatment of biliary and pancreatic ascariasis (25,107). Worms can be demonstrated as a linear defect within the pancreatic duct (Fig. 4.41) and may be removed endoscopically with a tripod device.

## Sphincter of Oddi dysfunction

Sphincter of Oddi dysfunction is a functional motor disorder that may result in a hypertonic sphincter with altered motility and impedance to the passage of bile and pancreatic secretion into the duodenum. This dysfunction may involve the major part of the sphincter of Oddi muscle segment or a smaller, more critical zone, the pancreatic duct segment. Consequently, impedance to pancreatic flow causes an increase in back pressure on pancreatic parenchyma leading to pancreatic cellular damage.

In adults, the leading cause of recurrent pancreatitis among patients previously given a diagnosis of idiopathic pancreatitis appears to be sphincter of Oddi dysfunction (18). It represents approximately 15% of patients with recurrent pancreatitis. Sphincter of Oddi manometry (108) constitutes the best diagnostic procedure and elevated sphincter of Oddi basal pressure (109), the major criterion, for diagnosis.

Guelrud *et al.* described 50 children with idiopathic recurrent pancreatitis in whom sphincter of Oddi dysfunction was demonstrated in three (6%) cases (25). Two of three children were treated by standard endoscopic sphincterotomy, with clinical improvement noted in one patient after a follow-up of 18 months. The third patient was treated by dual sphincterotomy of the pancreatic and common duct sphincters, after which the patient was markedly improved during the ensuing 4 years (110). Brown *et al.* found sphincter of Oddi dysfunction in three of 38 children (8%) with recurrent pancreatitis (111). Lemmel *et al.* studied 29 children with recurrent pancreatitis and found seven patients (24%) with sphincter of Oddi dysfunction (24). These patients are generally treated by conventional endoscopic sphincterotomy. However, not all patients had a good response presumably because with this treatment modality the pancreatic sphincter is not severed, and recurrent attacks of pancreatitis may be attributed to pancreatic sphincter dysfunction (112,113). A hypertensive pancreatic duct sphincter has been suggested as the cause of these recurrent episodes of pancreatitis (114). A subsequent endoscopic sphincterotomy of the pancreatic sphincter may be necessary to alleviate the problem. When symptoms are sufficient to warrant a therapeutic procedure, dual sphincterotomy of the pancreatic and biliary sphincters is generally favored (110). Failure to recognize dysfunction in both sphincters may result in incomplete therapy and persistence of symptoms. Greater experience will be necessary before firm recommendations can be made for optimal therapy.

# References


1. Hendren WH, Greep JM, Patton AS. Pancreatitis in childhood: experience with 15 cases. *Arch Dis Child* 1965; **40:** 132–45.
2. Jordan SC, Ament ME. Pancreatitis in children and adolescents. *J Pediatr* 1977; **91:** 211–6.
3. Ziegler DW, Long JA, Philippart AI, Klein MD. Pancreatitis in childhood: experience with 49 patients. *Ann Surg* 1988; **207:** 257–61.
4. Kattwinkel J, Lapey A, Di Sant'Agnese P, Edwards WA. Hereditary pancreatitis: three new kindred's and a critical review of the literature. *Pediatrics* 1973; **51:** 55–69.
5. Krauss RM, Levy AG. Subclinical chronic pancreatitis in type I hyperlipoproteinemia. *Am J Med* 1977; **62:** 144–9.

6.  Park RW, Grand RJ. Gastrointestinal manifestations of cystic fibrosis: a review. *Gastroenterology* 1981; **81:** 1143–61.

7.  Griffin M, Carey WD, Hermann R, Buonocore E. Recurrent acute pancreatitis and intussusception complicating an intraluminal duodenal diverticulum. *Gastroenterology* 1981; **81:** 345–8.

8.  Wagner CW, Golladay ES. Pancreas divisum and pancreatitis in children. *Am Surg* 1988; **54:** 22–6.

9.  Yaffe MR, Gutenberger JE. Chronic pancreatitis and pancreas divisum in an infant: diagnosed by endoscopic retrograde cholangiopancreatography and treated with somatostatin analog. *J Pediatr Gastroenterol Nutr* 1989; **9:** 108–11.

10.  Yedlin ST, Dubois RS, Philippart AI. Pancreas divisum. A cause of pancreatitis in childhood. *J Pediatr Surg* 1984; **19:** 793–94.

11.  Van Der Spuy S. Endoscopic retrograde cholangiopancreatography (ERCP) in children. *Endoscopy* 1978; **10:** 173–5.

12.  Werlin SL. Endoscopic retrograde cholangiopancreatography in children. *Gastrointest Endosc Clin North Am* 1994; **1:** 161–75.

13.  Agrawall RM, Brodmerkel GJ. Choledochal cyst presenting as pancreatitis. *Am J Gastroenterol* 1979; **71:** 408–11.

14.  Black PR, Welch KJ, Eraklis AJ. Juxtapancreatic intestinal duplications with pancreatic ductal communication: a cause of pancreatitis and recurrent abdominal pain in childhood. *J Pediatr Surg* 1986; **21:** 257–61.

15.  Lavine JE, Harrison M, Heyman MB. Gastrointestinal duplications causing relapsing pancreatitis in children. *Gastroenterology* 1989; **97:** 1556–58.

16.  Komura J, Yano H, Tanaka Y, *et al.* Annular pancreas associated with pancreaticobiliary maljunction in an infant. *Eur J Pediatr Surg* 1993; **3:** 244–7.

17.  Guelrud, M. Endoscopic retrograde cholangiopancreatography in the infant. In: Barkin J, O'Phelan CA, eds. *Advanced Therapeutic Endoscopy.* New York: Raven Press, 1990: 335–54.

18.  Venu RP, Geenen JE, Hogan W, Stone J, Johnson GK, Soergel K. Idiopathic recurrent pancreatitis. An approach to diagnosis and treatment. *Dig Dis Sci* 1989; **34:** 56–60.

19.  Forbes A, Leung JWC, Cotton PB. Relapsing acute and chronic pancreatitis. *Arch Dis Child* 1984; **59:** 927–34.

20.  Buckley A, Connon JJ. The role of ERCP in children and adolescents. *Gastrointest Endosc* 1990; **36:** 369–72.

21.  Putnam PE, Kocoshis SA, Orenstein SR, Schade RR. Pediatric endoscopic retrograde cholangiopancreatography. *Am J Gastroenterol* 1991; **86:** 824–30.

22.  Dité P, Vacek E, Stefan H, Koudelka J, Pozler O, Králová M. Endoscopic retrograde cholangiopancreatography in childhood. *Hepatogastroenterol* 1992; **39:** 291–3.

23.  Brown KO, Goldschmiedt M. Endoscopic therapy of biliary and pancreatic disorders in children. *Endoscopy* 1994; **26:** 719–23.

24.  Lemmel T, Hawes R, Sherman S, *et al.* Endoscopic evaluation and therapy of recurrent pancreatitis and pancreaticobiliary pain in the pediatric population. *Gastrointest Endosc* 1994; **40:** A54.

25.  Guelrud M, Mujica C, Jaen D, Plaz J, Arias J. The role of ERCP in the diagnosis and treatment of idiopathic recurrent pancreatitis in children and adolescents. *Gastrointest Endosc* 1994; **40:** 428–36.

26.  Beshlian K, Ryan JA. Pancreatitis in teenagers. *Am J Surg* 1986; **152:** 133–8.

27.  Karjoo M, Bishop H, Borns P, *et al.* Choledochal cyst presenting as recurrent pancreatitis. *Pediatrics* 1973; **51:** 289–91.

28. Taylor R, Auldist A. Choledochal cyst presenting as acute pancreatitis. *Aust N Z Surg* 1985; **55:** 611–2.

29. Shirai Z, Toriya H, Maeshiro K, Ikeda S. The usefulness of endoscopic retrograde cholangiopancreatography in infants and small children. *Am J Gastroenterol* 1993; **88:** 536–41.

30. Greene FL, Brown JJ, Rubinstein P, Anderson MC. Choledochocele and recurrent pancreatitis. Diagnosis and surgical management. *Am J Surg* 1985; **149:** 306–9.

31. Marshall JB, Halpin TC. Choledochocele as the cause of recurrent obstructive jaundice in childhood: diagnosis by ERCP. *Gastrointest Endosc* 1982; **28:** 88–90.

32. Venu RP, Geenen JE, Hogan WJ, Dodds WJ, Wilson SW, Stewart ET, Soergel KH. Role of endoscopic retrograde cholangiopancreatography in the diagnosis and treatment of choledochocele. *Gastroenterology* 1984; **87:** 1144–9.

33. Kagiyama S, Okazaki K, Yamamoto Y, Yamamoto Y. Anatomic variants of choledochocele and manometric measurements of pressure in the cele and the orifice zone. *Am J Gastroenterol* 1987; **82:** 641–9.

34. Guelrud M. Papillary stenosis. *Endoscopy* 1988; **20:** 193–202.

35. Guelrud M, Mendoza S, Viera L, Gelrud D. Somatostatin prevents acute pancreatitis after pancreatic duct sphincter hydrostatic balloon dilation in patients with idiopathic recurrent pancreatitis. *Gastrointest Endosc* 1991; **37:** 44–7.

36. Siegel JH, Harding GT, Chateau F. Endoscopic incision of choledochal cysts (choledochocele). *Endoscopy* 1981; **13:** 200–2.

37. Karp MP, Jewett TC, Cooney DR. Chronic relapsing pancreatitis in childhood caused by pancreaticobiliary ductal anomaly. *J Pediatr Gastroenterol Nutr* 1983; **2:** 324–8.

38. Mori K, Nagakawa T, Ohta T, *et al.* Acute pancreatitis associated with anomalous union of the pancreaticobiliary ductal system. *J Clin Gastroenterol* 1991; **13:** 673–7.

39. Gibson LE, Haller JA. Acute pancreatitis associated with congenital cyst of the common bile duct. *J Pediatr* 1959; **55:** 650–7.

40. Raffensperger BG, Given GZ, Warner RA. Fusiform dilatation of the common bile duct with pancreatitis. *J Pediatr Surg* 1973; **8:** 907–10.

41. Suda K, Miyano T, Konuma I, Matsumoto M. An abnormal pancreatico-choledocho ductal junction in cases of biliary tract carcinoma. *Cancer* 1983; **52:** 2086–88.

42. Cooperman AM, Sivak MV, Sullivan BH, Hermann RE. Endoscopic pancreatography: its value in preoperative and postoperative assessment of pancreatic disease. *Am J Surg* 1975; **129:** 38–43.

43. Cooperman M, Ferrara JJ, Carey LC. Thomas FB, Martin EW, Fromkes JJ. Idiopathic acute pancreatitis: the value of endoscopic retrograde cholangiopancreatography. *Surgery* 1981; **90:** 666–70.

44. Yatto RP, Siegel JH. Variant pancreatography. *Am J Gastroenterol* 1983; **78:** 115–8.

45. Sigfusson BF, Wehlin L, Lindstrom CG. Variants of pancreatic duct system of importance in endoscopic retrograde cholangiopancretography. Observations on autopsy specimens. *Acta Radiol Diag* 1983; **24:** 113–28.

46. Tulassay Z, Papp J, Farkas IE. Diagnostic aspects of incomplete pancreas divisum. *Gastrointest Endosc* 1986; **32:** 482.

47. Sugawa CH, Alexander JW, Nuñez DC, Matsuyama H. Pancreas divisum: is it a normal anatomic variant? *Am J Surg* 1987; **153:** 62–7.

48. Moreira VF, Meroño E, Ledo L, *et al.* Incomplete pancreas divisum. *Gastrointest Endosc* 1991; **37:** 104–5.

49. Guelrud M, Herrera I. Isolated ventral chronic pancreatitis in incomplete pancreas divisum and sphincter of Oddi dysfunction in an adolescent. *Gastrointest Endosc,* in press.

50. Fox VL, Lichtenstein DR, Carr-Locke DL. Incomplete pancreas divisum in children with recurrent pancreatitis. *Gastrointest Endosc* 1995; **41:** 337 (A).

51. Cotton PB. Congenital anomaly of pancreas divisum as a cause of obstructive pain and pancreatitis. *Gut* 1980; **21:** 105–14.

52. Satterfield ST, Mc Carthy JH, Geenen JE. Hogan NJ, Venu RP, Dodds NJ, Johnson GK. Clinical experience with pancreas divisum: preliminary results of manometry and endoscopic therapy. *Pancreas* 1988; **3:** 248–53.

53. Bernard JP, Sahel J, Giovanni M, Sarles H. Pancreas divisum is a probable cause of acute pancreatitis: a report of 137 cases. *Pancreas* 1990; **5:** 248–54.

54. Guelrud M. The incidence of pancreas divisum in children. *Gastrointest Endosc* 1996; **43:** 83–4.

55. Liguory C, Lefebvre JF, Carrard JM, Bonnel D, Fritsch J, Etienne JP. Le pancreas divisum: etude clinique et therapeutique chez l'homme: a propos de 87 cas. *Gastroenterol Clin Biol* 1986; **10:** 820–5.

56. Gregg JA. Pancreas divisum: its association with pancreatitis. *Am J Surg* 1977; **134:** 539–43.

57. Richter JM, Shapiro RH, Mulley AG, Warshaw AL. Association of pancreas divisum and pancreatitis, and its treatment by sphincterotomy of the accessory ampulla. *Gastroenterology* 1981; **81:** 1104–10.

58. Rosch W, Koch H, Schaffner O, Demling L. The clinical significance of pancreas divisum. *Gastrointest Endosc* 1976; **22:** 206–7.

59. Mitchell CJ, Lintott DJ, Ruddell WSJ, *et al.* Clinical relevance of an unfused pancreatic duct system. *Gut* 1979; **20:** 1066–71.

60. Delhaye M, Engelholm L, Cremer M. Pancreas divisum: congenital anatomic variant or anomaly? Contribution of endoscopic retrograde dorsal pancreatography. *Gastroenterology* 1985; **89:** 951–8.

61. Cotton PB. Pancreas divisum. Curiosity or culprit? *Gastroenterology* 1985; **89:** 1431–5.

62. Staritz M, Meyer KH. Elevated pressure in the dorsal part of pancreas divisum: the cause of chronic pancreatitis? *Pancreas* 1988; **3:** 108–10.

63. Warshaw AL, Richter JM, Schapiro RH. The cause and treatment of pancreatitis associated with pancreas divisum. *Am Surg* 1983; **198:** 443–52.

64. O'Connor KW, Lehman GA. An improved technique for accessory papilla cannulation in pancreas divisum. *Gastrointest Endosc* 1985; **31:** 13–7.

65. Rusnak CH, Hosie RT, Kuechler PM, McHattie JD, Piercey JR, Cameron RD. Pancreatitis associated with pancreas divisum: results of surgical intervention. *Am J Surg* 1988; **155:** 641–3.

66. Warshaw AL, Simeone J, Schapiro RH, Hedberg SE, Mueller PE, Ferrucci JT, Jr. Objective evaluation of ampullary stenosis with ultrasonography and pancreatic stimulation. *Am J Surg* 1985; **149:** 65–72.

67. Lowes JR, Lees WR, Cotton PB. Pancreatic duct dilatation after secretin stimulation in patients with pancreas divisum. *Pancreas* 1989; **4:** 371–4.

68. Eisen G, Schutz S, Metzler D, Baillie J, Cotton PB. Santorinicele: new evidence for obstruction in pancreas divisum. *Gastrointest Endosc* 1994; **40:** 73–6.

69. Blair AJ, Russell CG, Cotton PB. Resection for pancreatitis in patients with pancreas divisum. *Ann Surg* 1984; **200:** 590–4.

70. Benage D, McHenry R, Hawes RH, O'Connor KW, Lehman GA. Minor papilla cannulation and dorsal ductography in pancreas divisum. *Gastrointest Endosc* 1990; **36:** 553–7.

71. Warshaw AL, Simeone JF, Schapiro RH, Flavin-Warshaw B. Evaluation and treatment of the dominant dorsal duct syndrome (pancreas divisum redefined). *Am J Surg* 1990; **159:** 59–64.

72. Keith RG, Shapero TF, Saibil FG, Moore TL. Dorsal duct sphincterotomy is effective long-term treatment of acute pancreatitis associated with pancreas divisum. *Surgery* 1989; **106:** 660–7.

73. Madura JA. Pancreas divisum: stenosis of the dorsally dominant duct. A surgically correctable lesion. *Am J Surg* 1986; **151:** 742–5.

74. Siegel JH, Pullano W, Ben-Zvi JS, Cooperman AM. Effectiveness of endoscopic drainage for pancreas divisum. *Endoscopy* 1990; **20:** 129–32.

75. Cotton PB. Duodenoscopic papillotomy at the minor papilla of Vater for recurrent dorsal pancreatitis. *Endosc Dig* 1978; **3:** 27–8.

76. Soehendra N, Kempeneers I, Nam VC, Grimm H. Endoscopic dilatation and papillotomy of the accessory papilla and internal drainage in pancreas divisum. *Endoscopy* 1986; **18:** 129–32.

77. Lehman GA, Sherman S, Nisi R, Hawes RH. Pancreas divisum: results of minor papilla sphincterotomy. *Gastrointest Endosc* 1993; **39:** 1–8.

78. Chevillote G, Sahel J, Pietri H, Sarles H. Recurrent acute pancreatitis associated with pancreas divisum. A clinical study of 12 cases. *Gastroenterol Clin Biol* 1984; **8:** 352–8.

79. Dunham F, Delteure M, Jeanmart T, Toussaint J, Cremer M. Special catheters for ERCP. *Endoscopy* 1981; **13:** 81–5.

80. Elmore MF, Lehman GA, Meadows JR. Endoscopic retrograde cannulation of the accessory papilla. *Gastrointest Endosc* 1987; **23:** 170.

81. Adzick NS, Shamberger RC, Winter HS, Hendren WH. Surgical treatment of pancreas divisum causing pancreatitis in children. *J Pediatr Surg* 1989; **24:** 54–8.

82. Siegel JH, Guelrud M. Endoscopic cholangiopancreatoplasty: hydrostatic balloon dilation in the bile duct and pancreas. *Gastrointest Endosc* 1983; **29:** 99–103.

83. McCarthy J, Geenen JE, Hogan WJ. Preliminary experience with endoscopic stent placement in benign pancreatic diseases. *Gastrointest Endosc* 1988; **34:** 16–8.

84. Lans JI, Geenen JE, Johanson JF, Hogan WJ. Endoscopic therapy in patients with pancreas divisum and acute pancreatitis: a prospective, randomized, controlled clinical trial. *Gastrointest Endosc* 1992; **38:** 430–4.

85. Coleman SD, Eisen GM, Throughton AB, Cotton PB. Endoscopic treatment in pancreas divisum. *Am J Gastroenterol* 1994; **89:** 1152–5.

86. Kozarek RA. Pancreatic stents can induce ductal changes consistent with chronic pancreatitis. *Gastrointest Endosc* 1990; **36:** 93–5.

87. Gulliver DJ, Edmunds S, Baker M, *et al.* Stent placement for benign pancreatic disease: correlation between ERCP findings and clinical response. *Am J Roent* 1992; **159:** 751–5.

88. Sherman S, Alvarez C, Robert M, *et al.* Polyethylene pancreatic duct stent-induced changes in the normal dog pancreas. *Gastrointest Endosc* 1993; **39:** 658–64.

89. Stofer BE. Annular pancreas: a tabulation of the recent literature and report of a case. *Am J Med Sci* 1944; **207:** 430–5.

90. Yogi Y, Shibue T, Hashimoto S. Annular pancreas detected in adults, diagnosed by endoscopic retrograde cholangiopancreatography: report of four cases. *Gastroenterol Jpn* 1987; **22:** 92–9.

91. Lehman GA, Oçonnor KW. Coexistence of annular pancreas and pancreas divisum. ERCP diagnosis. *Gastrointest Endosc* 1985; **31:** 25–8.

92. Lechner GW, Read RC. Agenesis of the dorsal pancreas in an adult diabetic presenting with duodenal ileus. *Ann Surg* 1966; **163:** 311–4.

93. Gilinsky NH, Del Favero G, Cotton PB, Lees WR. Congenital short pancreas: a report of two cases. *Gut* 1985; **26:** 304–10.

94. Rosenstock F, Achkar E. A "short pancreas". *Gastrointest Endosc* 1986; **32:** 296–7.

95. Hadar H, Gadoth N, Herskowitz P, Heifetz M. Short pancreas and polysplenia syndrome. *Acta Radiol* 1991; **32:** 299–301.

96. Bretaque JF, Darnault P, Raoul JL, Gaudon Y, Gosselin M, Cousin P, Gastard J. Calcifying pancreatitis of a congenital short pancreas: a case report with successful endoscopic papillotomy. *Am J Gastroenterol* 1987; **82:** 1314–7.

97. Holstege A, Barner S, Brambs HJ, Wenz W, Gerok W, Farthmann EH. Relapsing pancreatitis associated with duodenal wall cysts. Diagnostic approach and treatment. *Gastroenterology* 1985; **88:** 814–9.

98. Kalvaria I, Bornman PC, Girdwood AH, Marks IN. Periampullary cyst: a surgical remediable cause of pancreatitis. *Gut* 1987; **28:** 358–62.

99. Nosher JL, Seaman WB. Association of intraluminal duodenal diverticulum with acute pancreatitis. *Radiology* 1975; **115:** 21–2.

100. Griffin M, Carey WD, Hermann R, Buonocore E. Recurrent acute pancreatitis and intussusception complicating an intraluminal duodenal diverticulum. *Gastroenterology* 1981; **81:** 345–8.

101. Viceconte G, Viceconte GW, Bogliolo G. Endoscopic manometry of the sphincter of Oddi in patients with and without yuxtapapillary duodenal diverticula. *Scand J Gastroenterol* 1984; **19:** 329–33.

102. Lauretta R, Plaz J, Rojas O, Villani D, Castillo J, Guelrud M. Divertículos duodenales yuxtapapilares. *Gen* 1988; **42:** 95–8.

103. Thomas E, Reddy KR. Cholangitis and pancreatitis due to yuxtapapillary duodenal diverticulum. Endoscopic sphincterotomy is the other alternative in selected cases. *Am J Gastroenterol* 1982; **77:** 303–4.

104. Johanson JF, Geenen JE, Hogan WJ, Huibregtse K. Endoscopic therapy of a duodenal duplication cyst. *Gastrointest Endosc* 1992; **38:** 60–4.

105. Krige JEJ, Lewis G, Bronman PC. Recurrent pancreatitis caused by calcified ascaris in the duct of Wirsung. *Am J Gastroenterol* 1987; **82:** 256–7.

106. Maddern GJ, Dennison AR, Blumgart LH. Fatal ascaris pancreatitis: an uncommon problem in the west. *Gut* 1992; **33:** 402–4.

107. Khuroo MS, Zargar SA, Yatoo GN, Javid G, Dar MY, Boda MI, Khan BA. Worm extraction and biliary drainage in hepatobiliary and pancreatic ascariasis. *Gastrointest Endosc* 1993; **39:** 38–46.

108. Guelrud M, Mendoza S, Rossiter G, Villegas MI. Sphincter of Oddi manometry in healthy volunteers. *Dig Dis Sci* 1990; **35:** 38–46.

109. Toouli J, Roberts-Thomson IC, Dent J, Lee J. Sphincter of Oddi motility disorders in patients with idiopathic recurrent pancreatitis. *Br J Surg* 1985; **72:** 859–63.

110. Guelrud M, Plaz J, Mendoza S, Beker B, Rojas O, Rossiter G. Endoscopic treatment in type II pancreatic sphincter dysfunction. *Gastrointest Endosc* 1995; **41:** (A)398.

111. Brown CW, Werlin SL, Geenen JE, Schmalz M. The diagnostic and therapeutic role of endoscopic retrograde cholangiopancreatography in children. *J Pediatr Gastroenterol Nut* 1993; **17:** 19–23.

112. Hogan WJ, Geenen JE, Kruidenier J. Effectiveness of conventional sphincteroplasty in relieving pancreatic duct sphincter pressure in patients with idiopathic recurrent pancreatitis. *Gastroenterology* 1983; **84:** A189.

113. Guelrud M, Siegel JH. Hypertensive pancreatic duct sphincter as a cause of pancreatitis. Successful treatment with hydrostatic balloon dilation. *Dig Dis Sci* 1984; **29:** 225–31.

114. Silverman WB, Ruffolo TA, Sherman S, Hawes RH, Lehman GA. Correlation of basal sphincter pressures measured from the bile duct and the pancreatic duct in patients with suspected sphincter of Oddi dysfunction. *Gastrointest Endosc* 1992; **38:** 440–3.

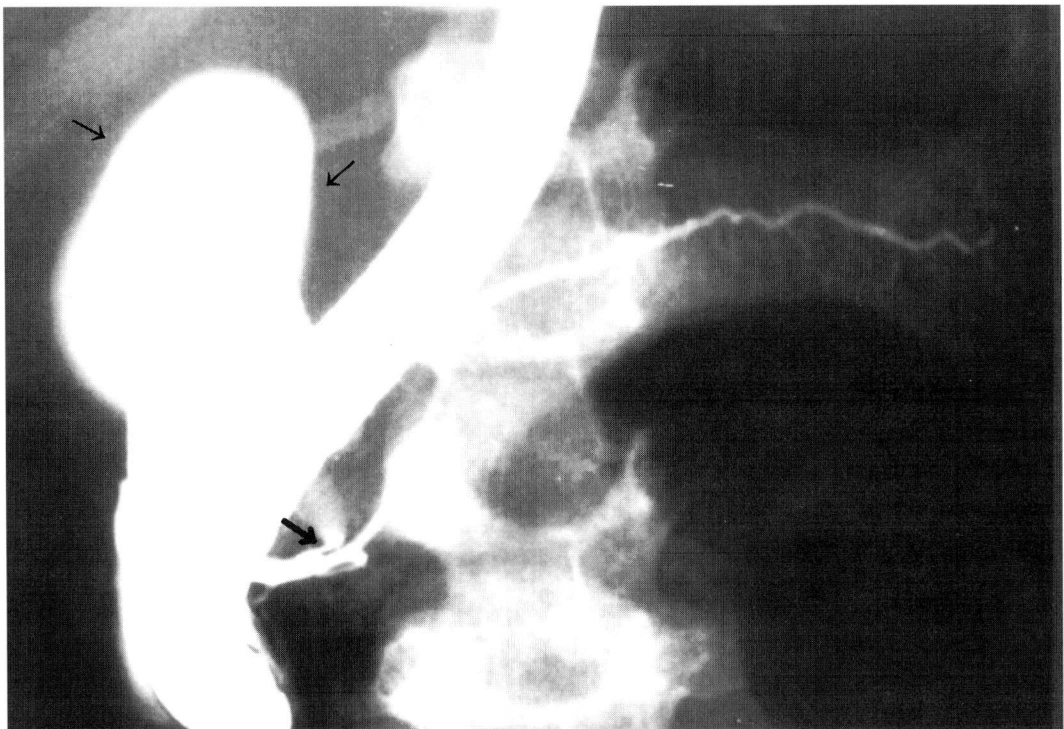

***Figure 4.1***

Choledochal cyst in a 4-year-old female with recurrent pancreatitis. Anomalous pancreaticobiliary union type BP configuration. Normal pancreatic duct. Type IA choledochal cyst (↑) with a stricture at the end of the common duct (↑).

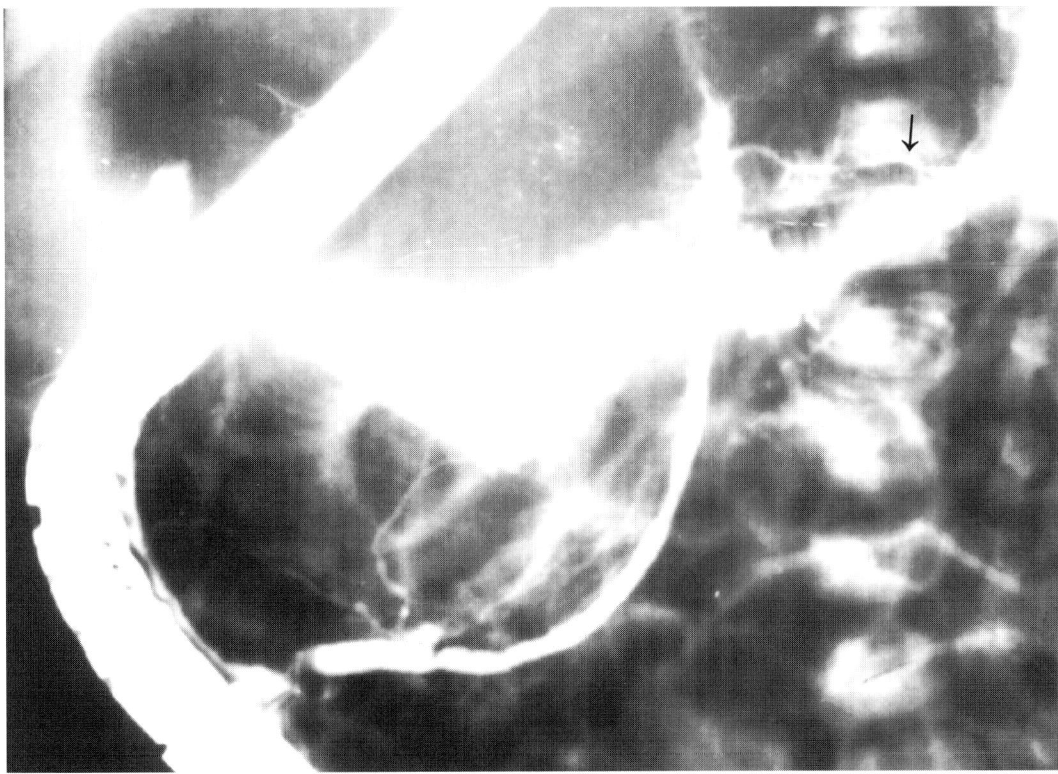

***Figure 4.2***

Choledochal cyst in a 1-year-old male infant with two attacks of acute pancreatitis. A gigantic choledochal cyst is not visualized. The pancreatic duct is abnormally long and dilated at the head and body of the pancreas. The tail of the pancreas is normal (↑).

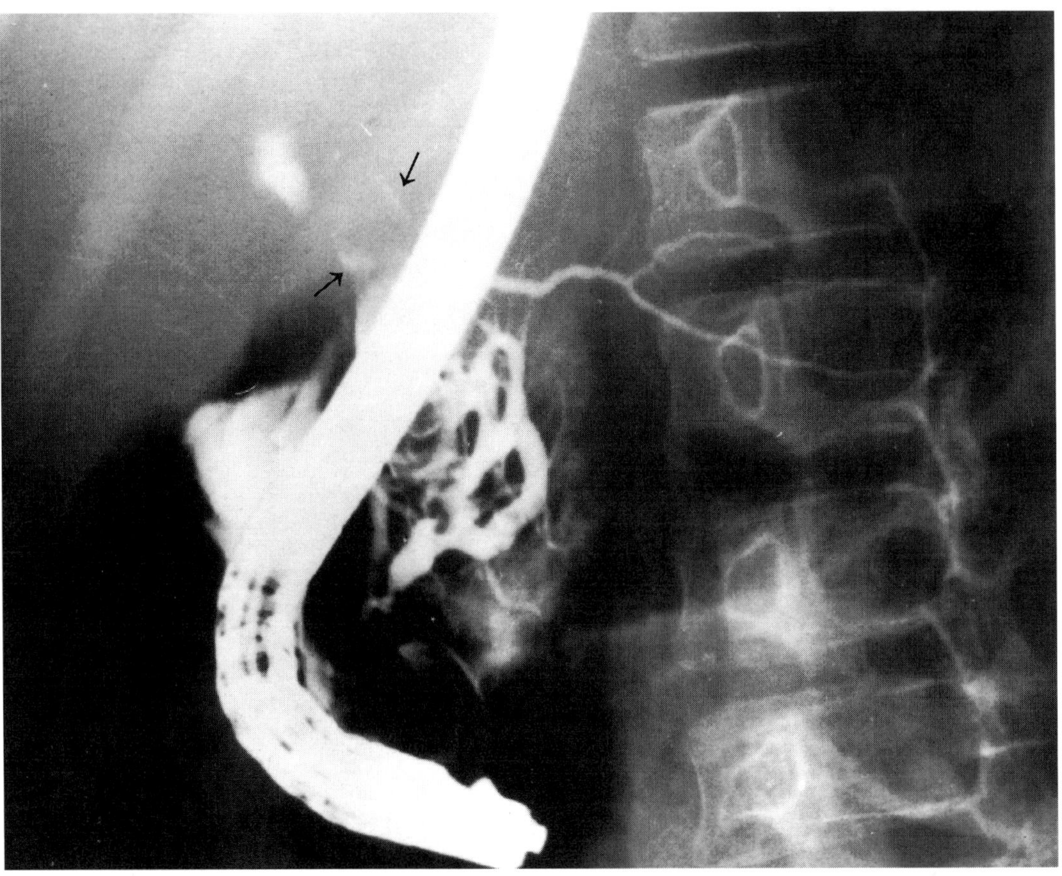

**Figure 4.3**
Choledochal cyst in a 14-year-old female with recurrent pancreatitis. Anomalous pancreaticobiliary union type BP configuration. The pancreatic duct and accessory duct are dilated and tortuous with dilated and irregular communicating branches. There is a bifurcation at the tail of the pancreas. A choledochal cyst (↑) is visualized with a stricture at the biliopancreatic junction.

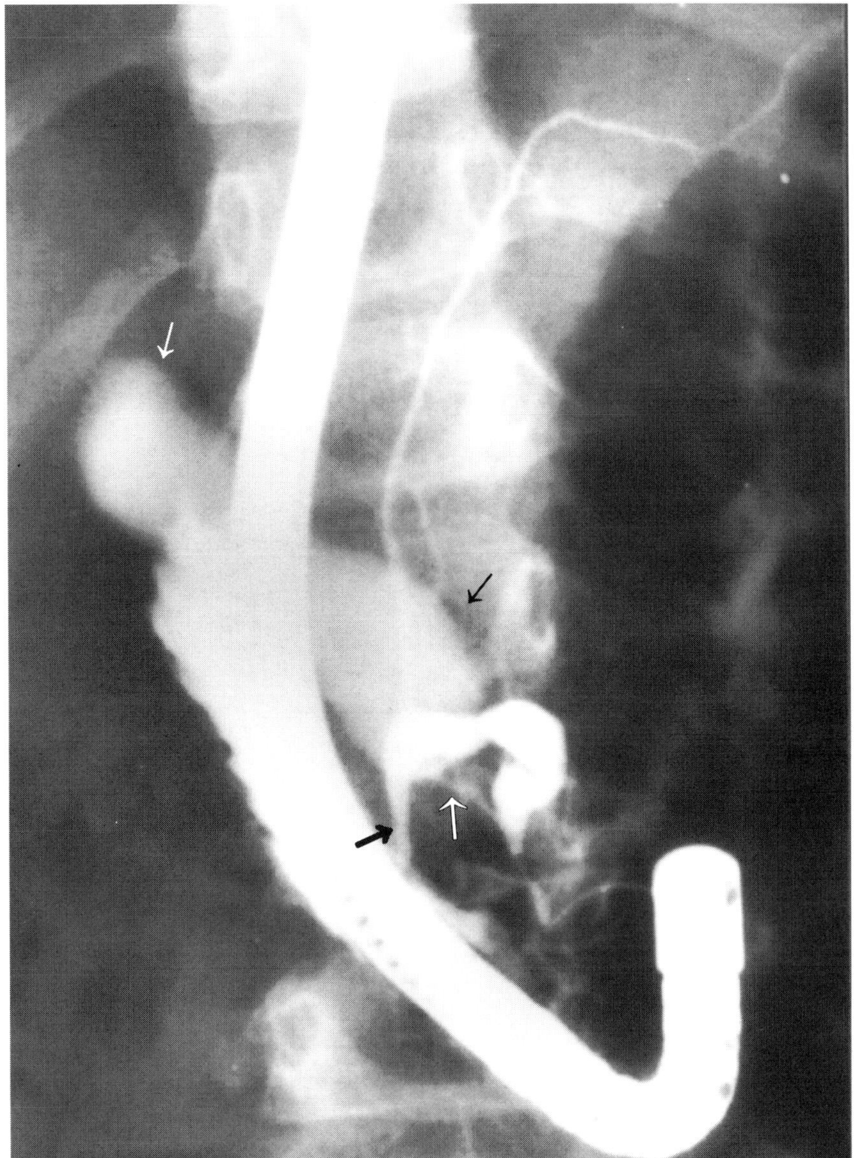

***Figure 4.4***
Choledochal cyst in a 16-year-old female with recurrent pancreatitis. Anomalous pancreaticobiliary union type BP configuration. Dilated pancreatic duct at the head of the pancreas. Dilated accessory duct. (↑) Normal pancreatic duct at the body and tail of the pancreas. Choledochal cyst Type IA (↑) with a long stricture (⇑) at the end of the common duct.

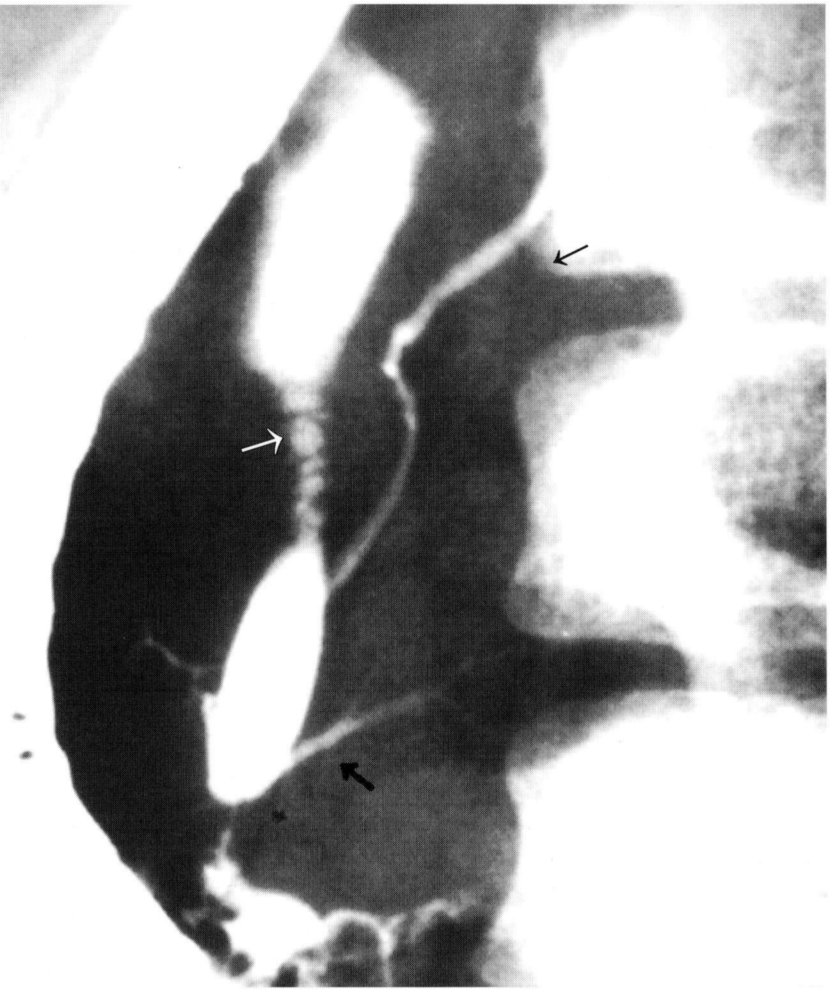

***Figure 4.5***
Choledochal cyst and pancreas divisum in a 4-year-old female with recurrent pancreatitis. Long dilated common channel. Normal ventral pancreas (↑). Dilated dorsal pancreatic duct (↑). Fusiform choledochal cyst (Type IC) with irregular stricture at the distal common duct (↑).

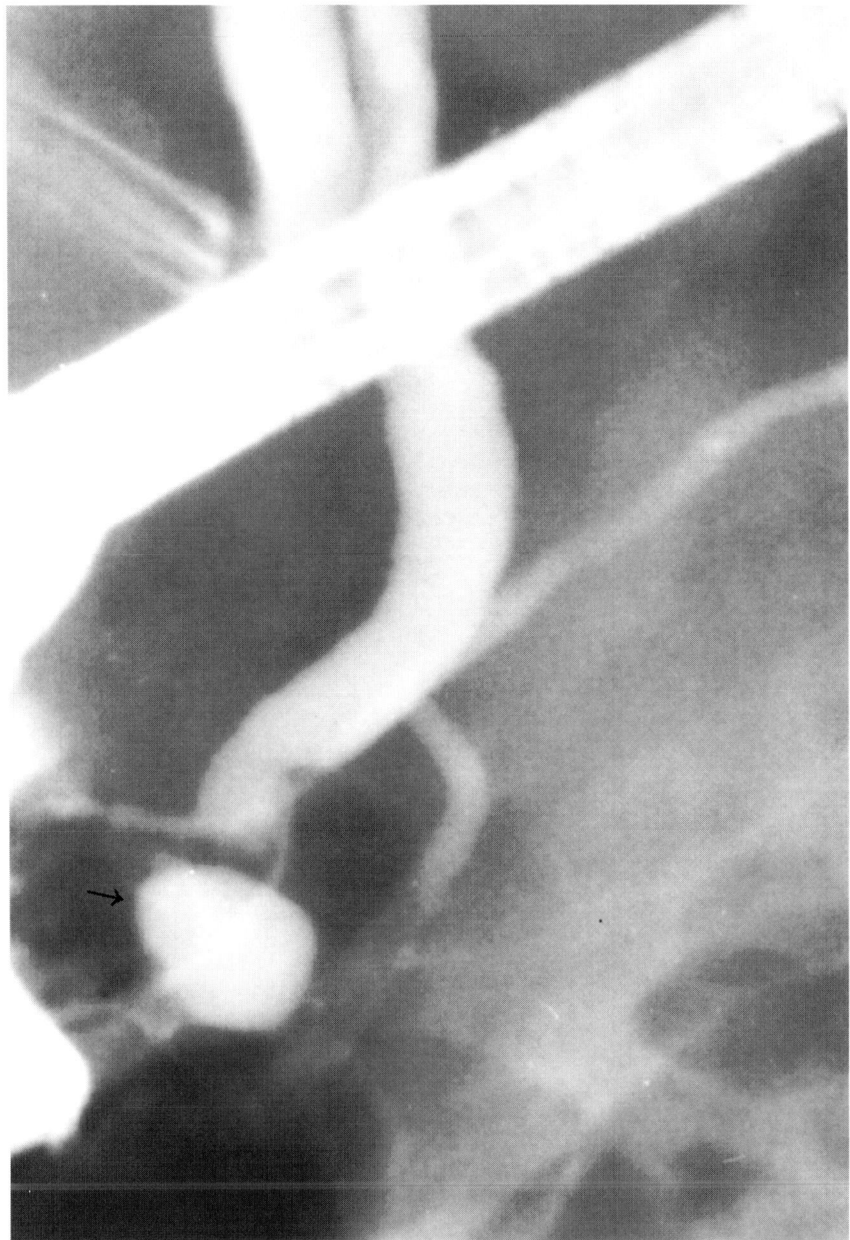

***Figure 4.6***
Choledochocele (Type III choledochal cyst) in a 18-year-old female with recurrent pancreatitis. Cystic dilatation at the common channel (↑). Dilated common duct and pancreatic duct. After endoscopic sphincterotomy, the patient remained asymptomatic for the ensuing 3 years.

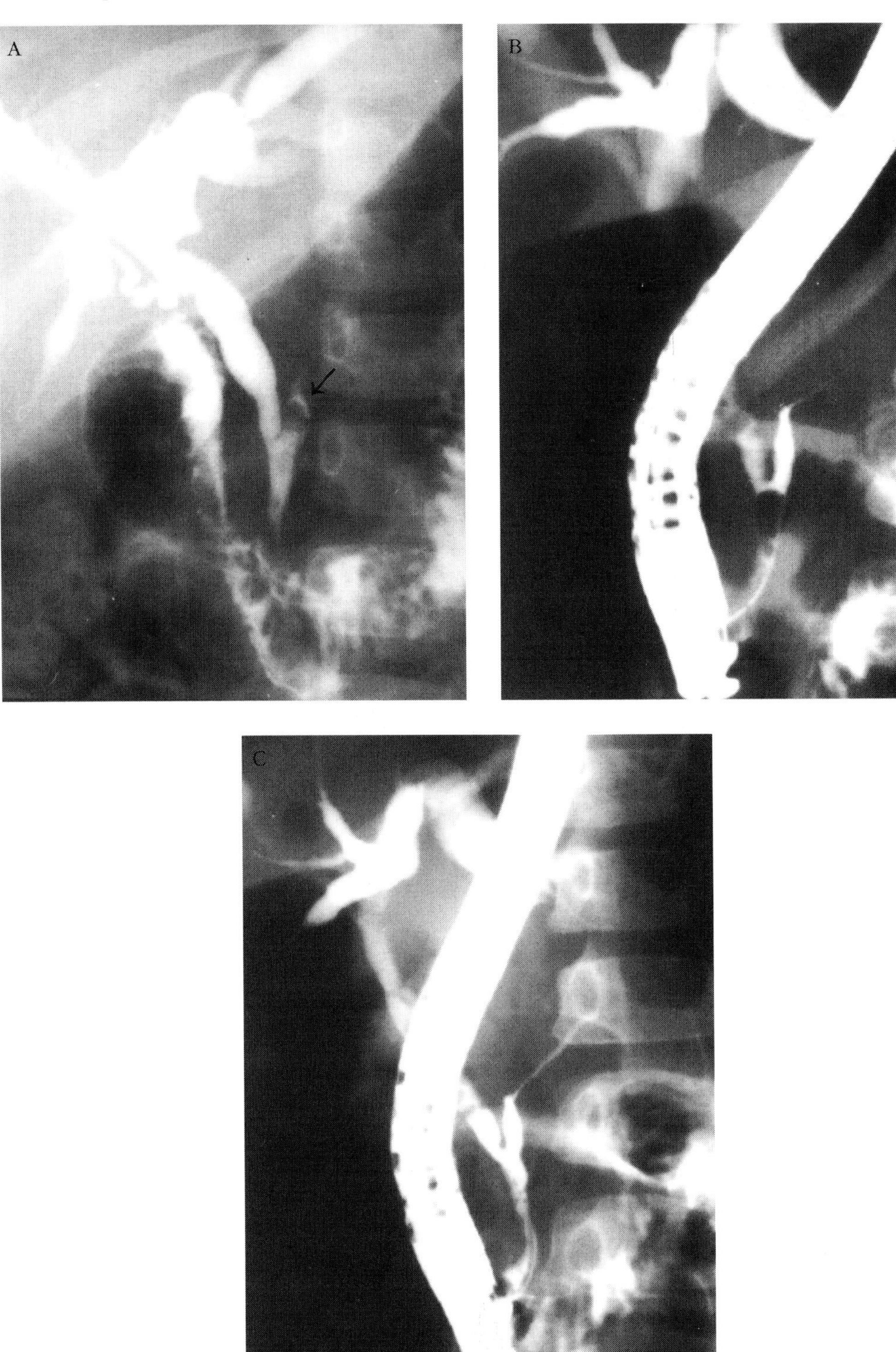

***Figure 4.7***
Choledochal cyst in a 6-year-old female with recurrent pancreatitis. (A) Anomalous pancreaticobiliary union type long "Y" configuration. Dilated pancreatic duct with a stone (↑). Cystic dilation of the entire biliary tree (Type IV A choledochal cyst). (B) After endoscopic sphincterotomy the pancreatic stone is removed with a Fogarty balloon. (C) The common channel orifice is widely open.

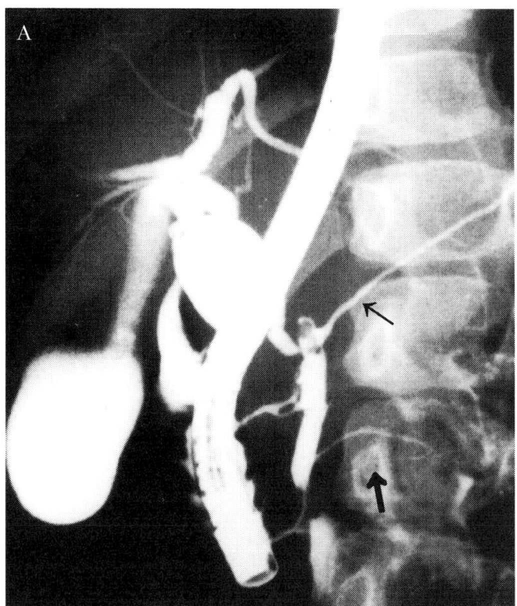 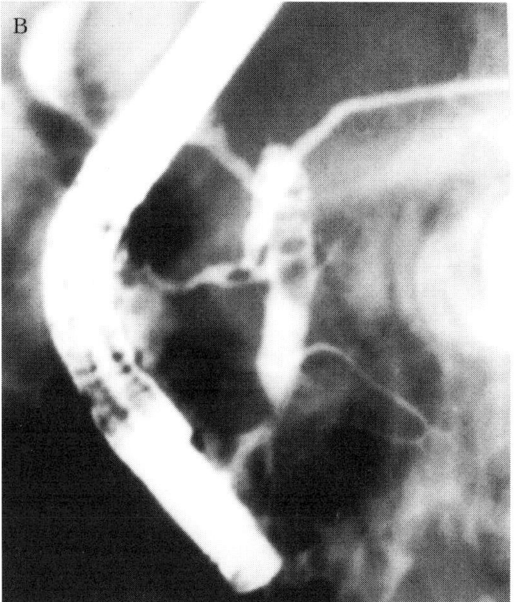

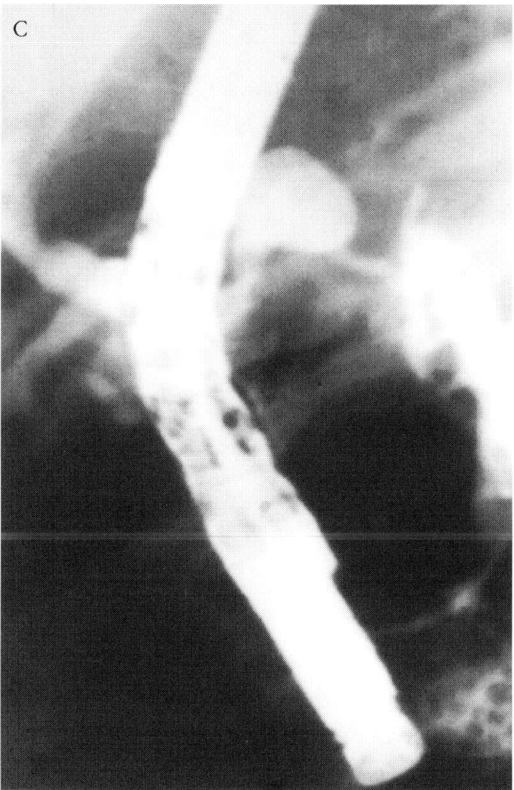

***Figure 4.8***

Choledochal cyst and pancreas divisum in a 5-year-old male with recurrent pancreatitis treated by endoscopic sphincterotomy. (A) Long common channel with a stone. Normal ventral pancreas (↑). Slightly dilated dorsal pancreas which communicates with the middle portion of the common duct (↑). Narrow stricture in the common duct. Typical cyst dilatation (Type IA choledochal cyst) of the common duct above the stricture. An endoscopic sphincterotomy with removal of a white, soft pancreatic stone, was performed. The patient remained symptom free during 5 years. (B) ERCP performed 5 years after cyst resection with hepatojejunostomy. In the last year, the patient had two attacks of acute pancreatitis. Duodenoscopy demonstrated a stenotic papillary orifice. A sphincterotomy was performed. A cholangiogram showed multiple common duct stones. (C) Multiple soft whitish stones were removed with a Fogarty balloon.

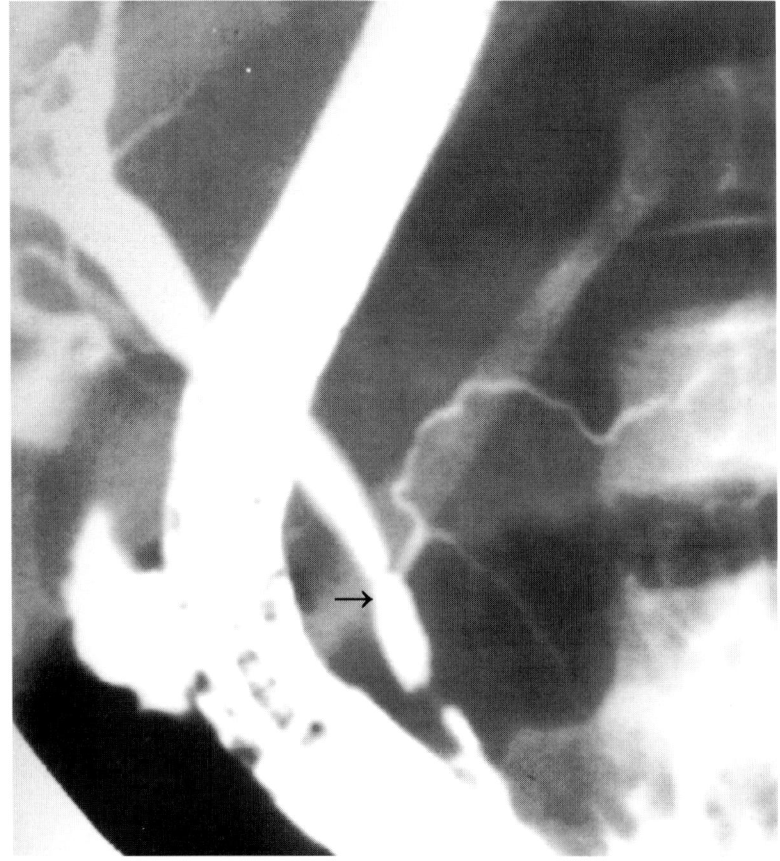

***Figure 4.9***
Anomalous pancreaticobiliary union type PB in a 5-year-old female with recurrent pancreatitis. Normal pancreatic duct. Annular stricture (↑) at the pancreaticobiliary union. (Courtesy of Todd H. Baron, MD., University of Alabama at Birmingham).

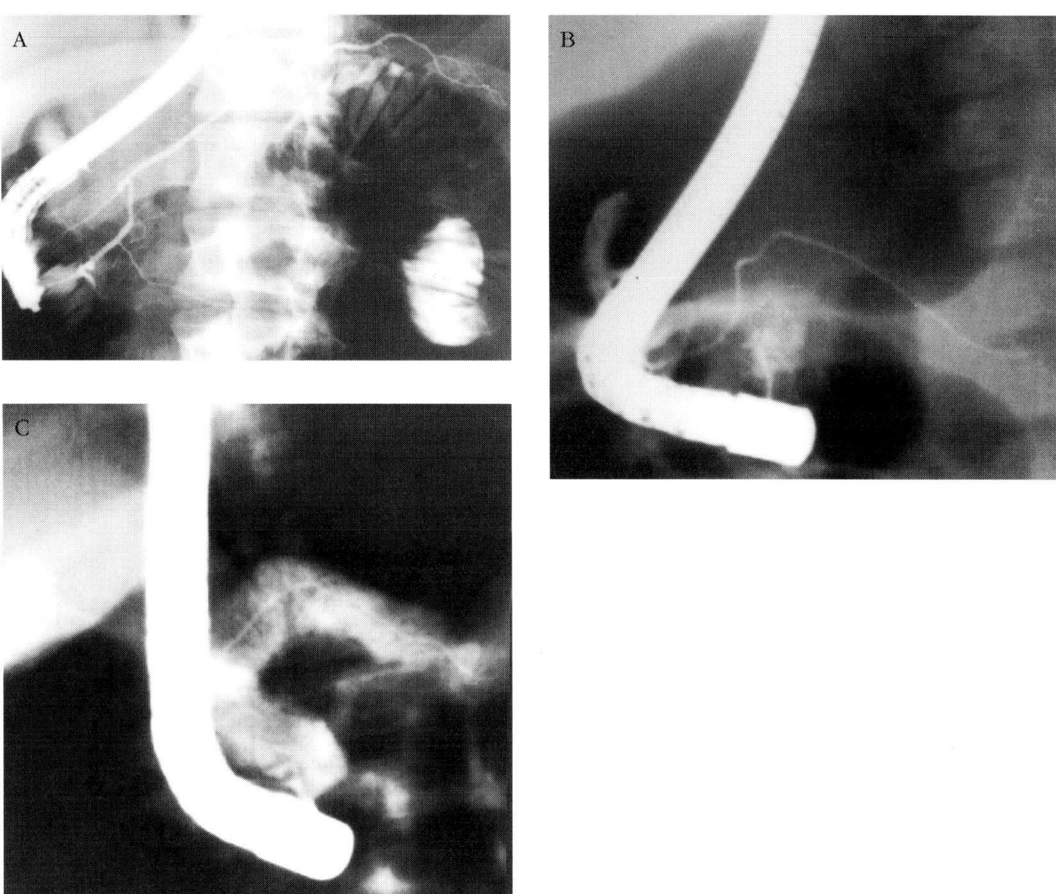

**_Figure 4.10_**
Normal pancreatic duct. (A) Normal pancreatic duct in a 14-year-old male. The accessory duct is located superior to the main pancreatic duct. The uncinate process branches are located inferior to the main pancreatic duct. (B) Normal pancreatic duct in a 2-month-old infant with biliary atresia. (C) Normal pancreatic duct with acinogram in a 26-day-old neonate with biliary atresia.

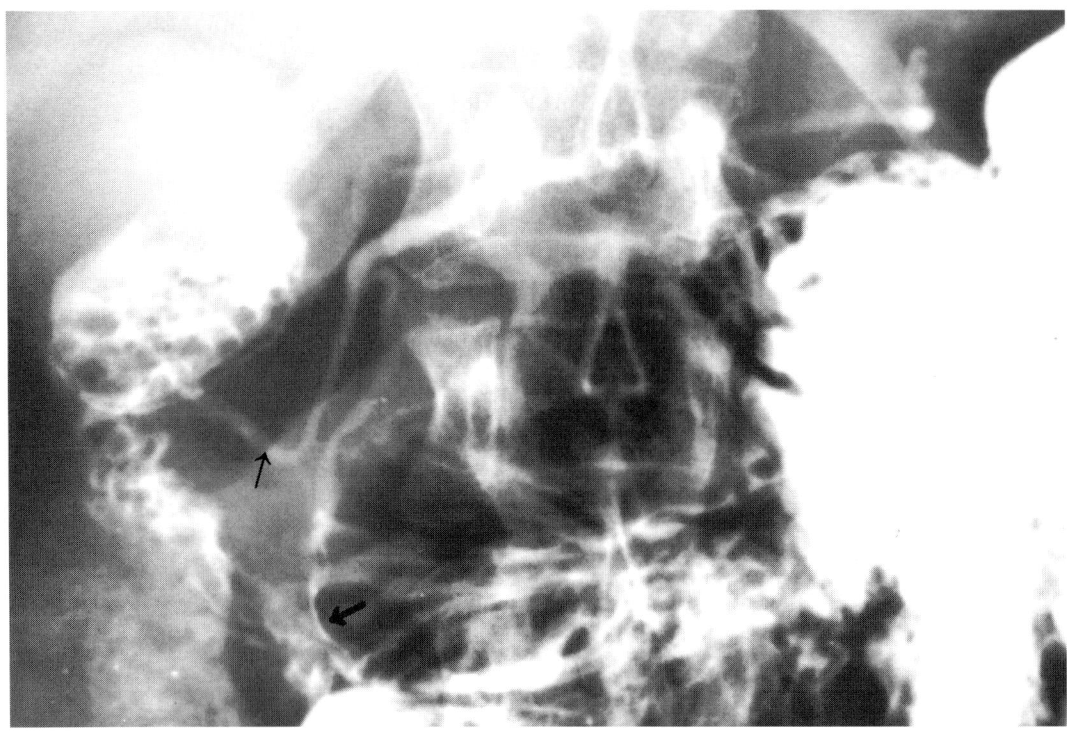

***Figure 4.11***
Abnormal location of the papilla. The accessory duct (↑) drains through the minor papilla located in the duodenal bulb. The main pancreatic duct enters the duodenum in the distal second portion (↑).

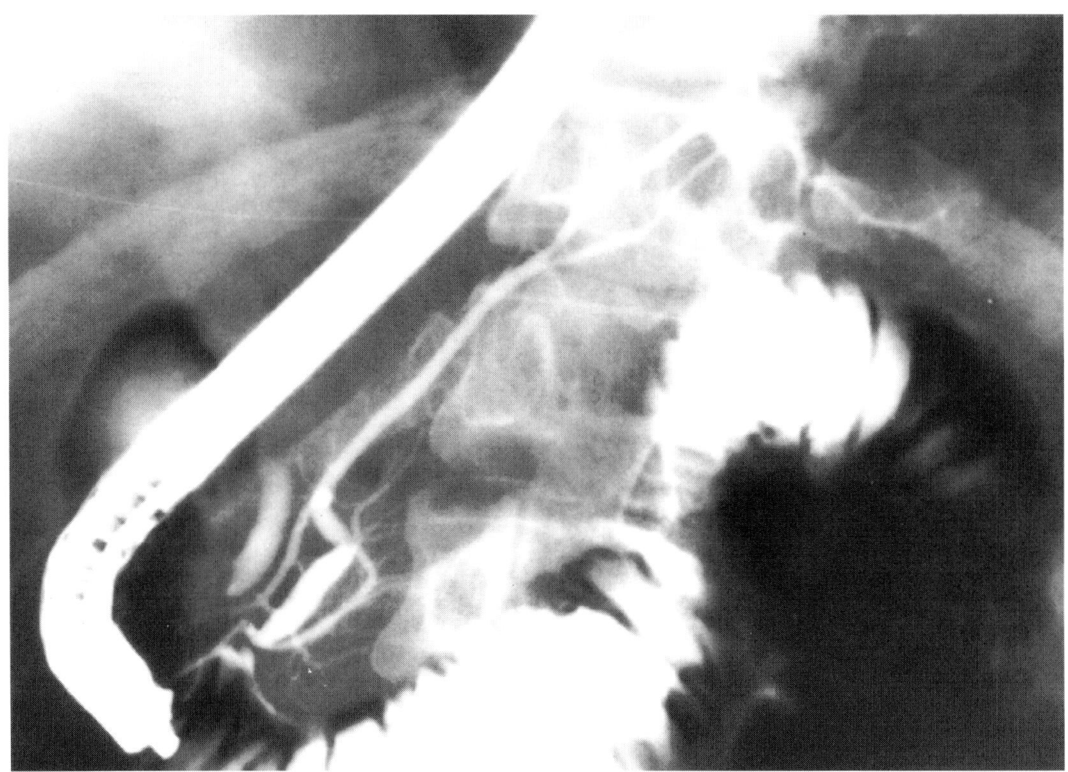

***Figure 4.12***
Bifurcation of the main pancreatic duct.

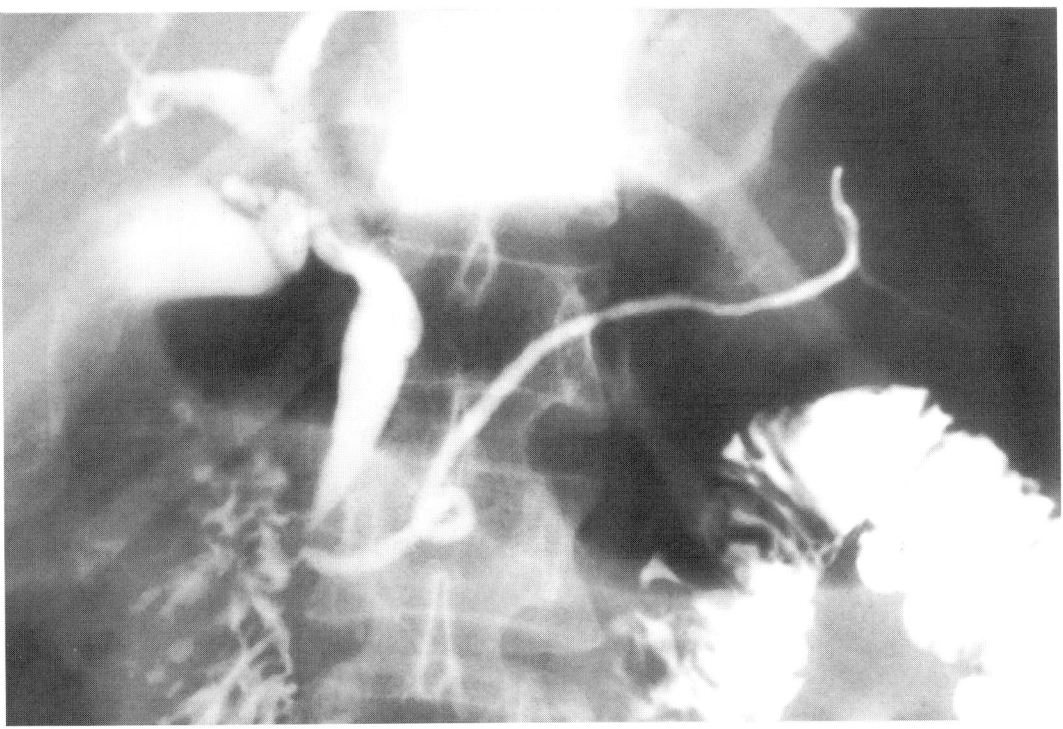

***Figure 4.13***
Loop in the pancreatic duct.

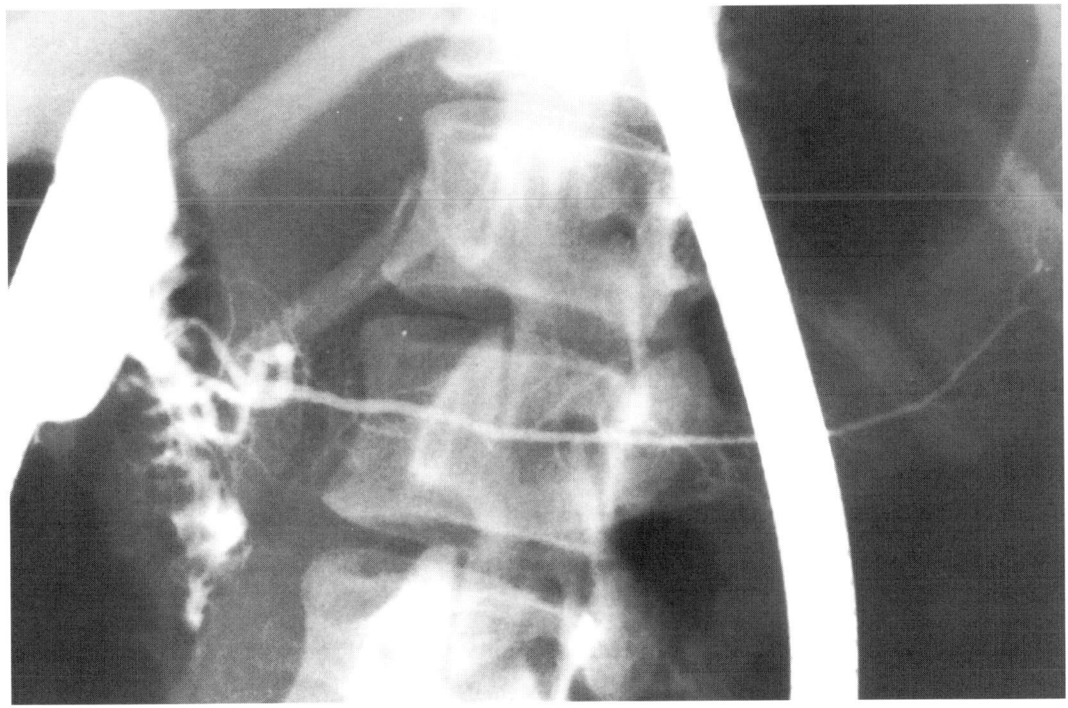

***Figure 4.14***
Double loop at the head of the pancreas. The pancreatic duct is opacified through the minor papilla.

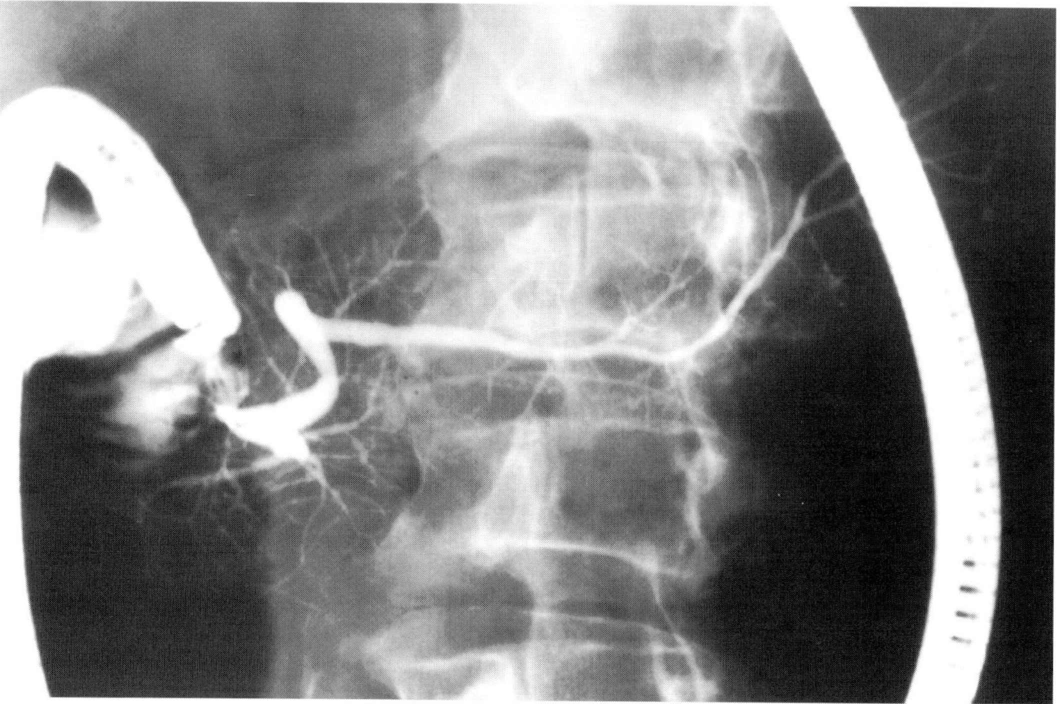

**Figure 4.15**
Acinarization of the entire pancreatic duct may simulate an enlarged pancreas.

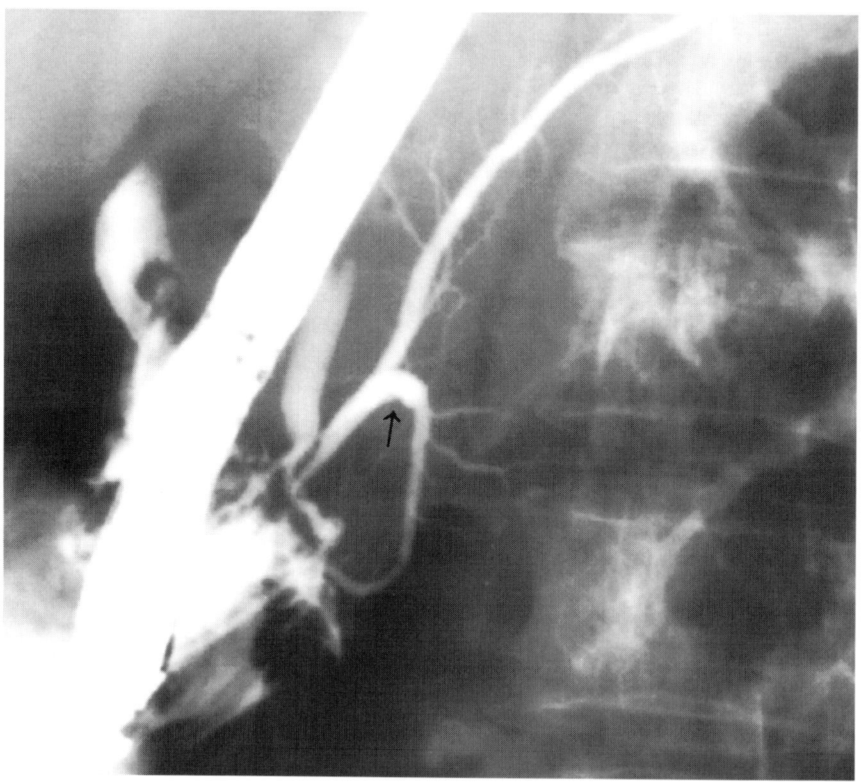

**Figure 4.16**
Prominent uncinate process of the pancreas. Anomalous pancreaticobiliary union type long
"Y". Dilated branch of the uncinate process (↑) with normal primary and secondary branches.

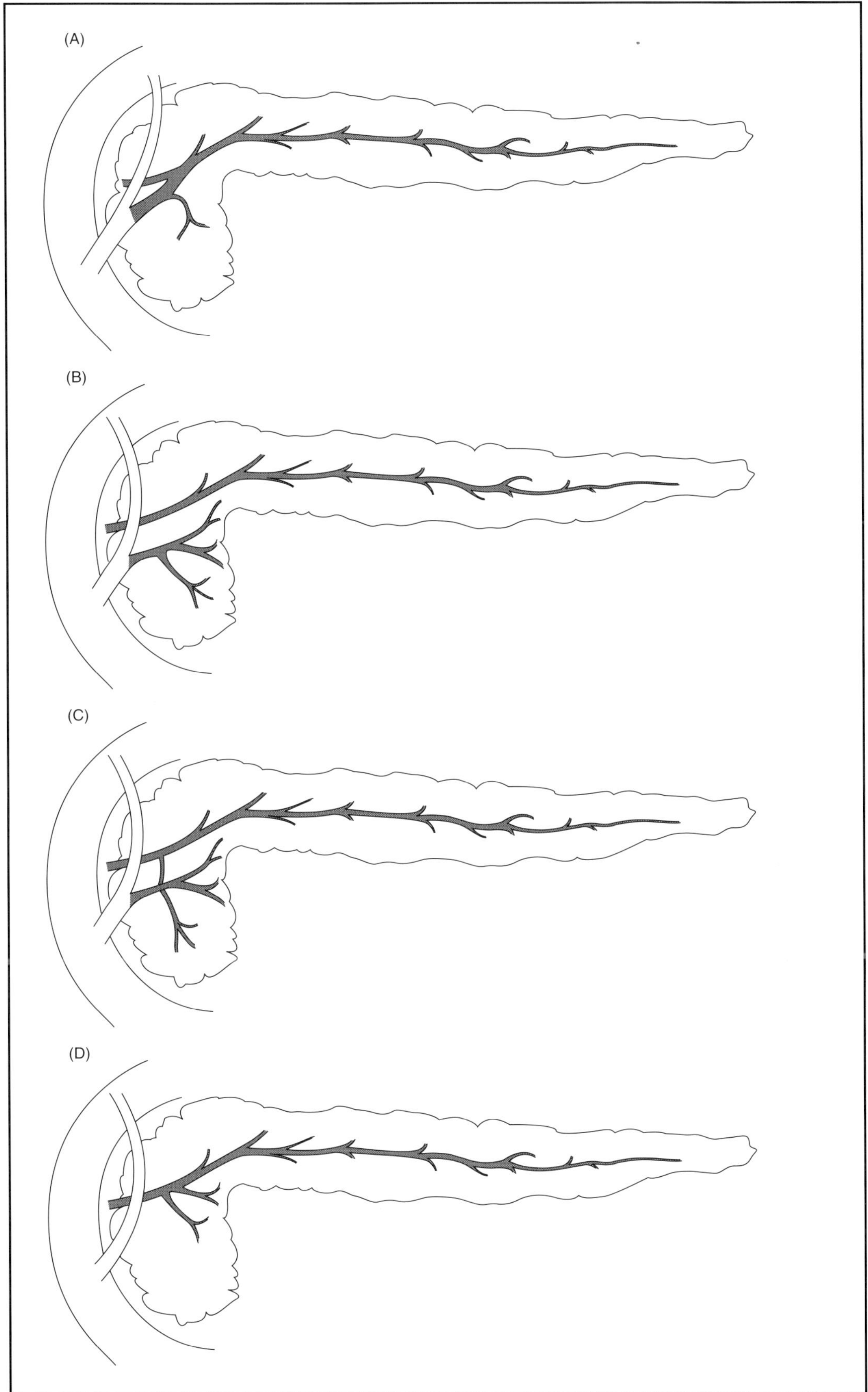


***Figure 4.17***

Schematic representation of pancreatic fusion anomalies. (A) Normal pancreatic fusion. (B) Pancreas divisum. (C) Incomplete pancreas divisum. (D) Absence of Wirsung duct.

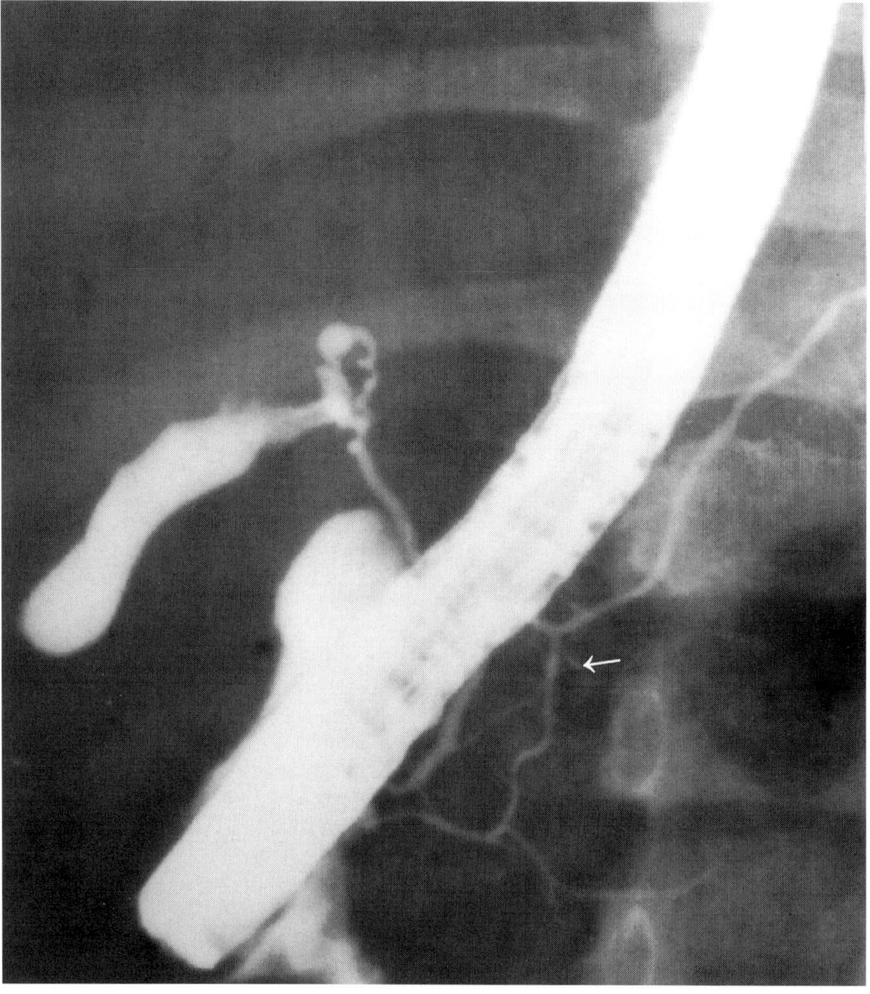

***Figure 4.18***

Incomplete pancreas divisum in a 2-month-old infant with biliary atresia. Filling of the ventral pancreatic duct. A communicating branch of the ventral pancreas (↑) joins the dorsal pancreas.

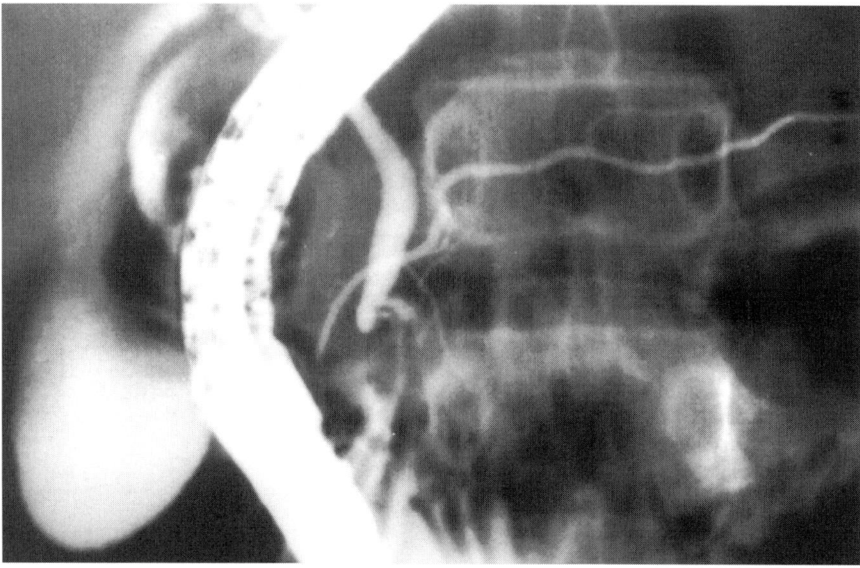

***Figure 4.19***

Incomplete pancreas divisum in a 10-year-old female with recurrent pancreatitis. Filling of the ventral pancreatic duct with branching of that system. Filling of the dorsal pancreatic duct (dominant Santorini) through a communicating branch.

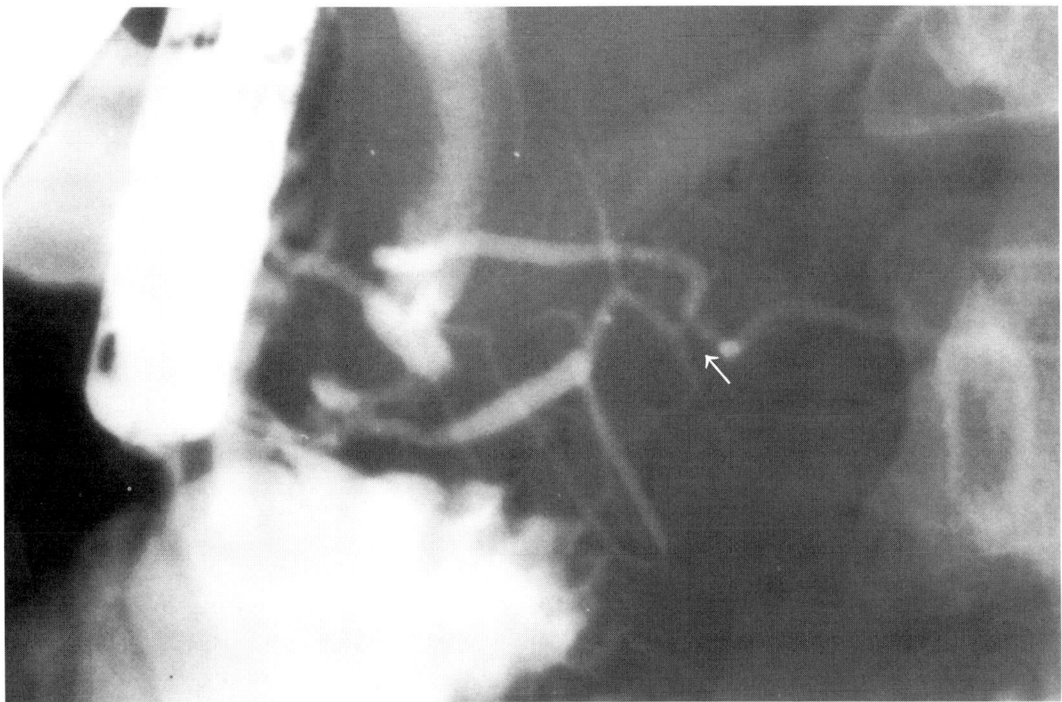

***Figure 4.20***
Incomplete pancreas divisum. Filling of the ventral pancreatic duct with branching of that system. A rudimentary branch (↑) opacifies the dorsal pancreatic duct.

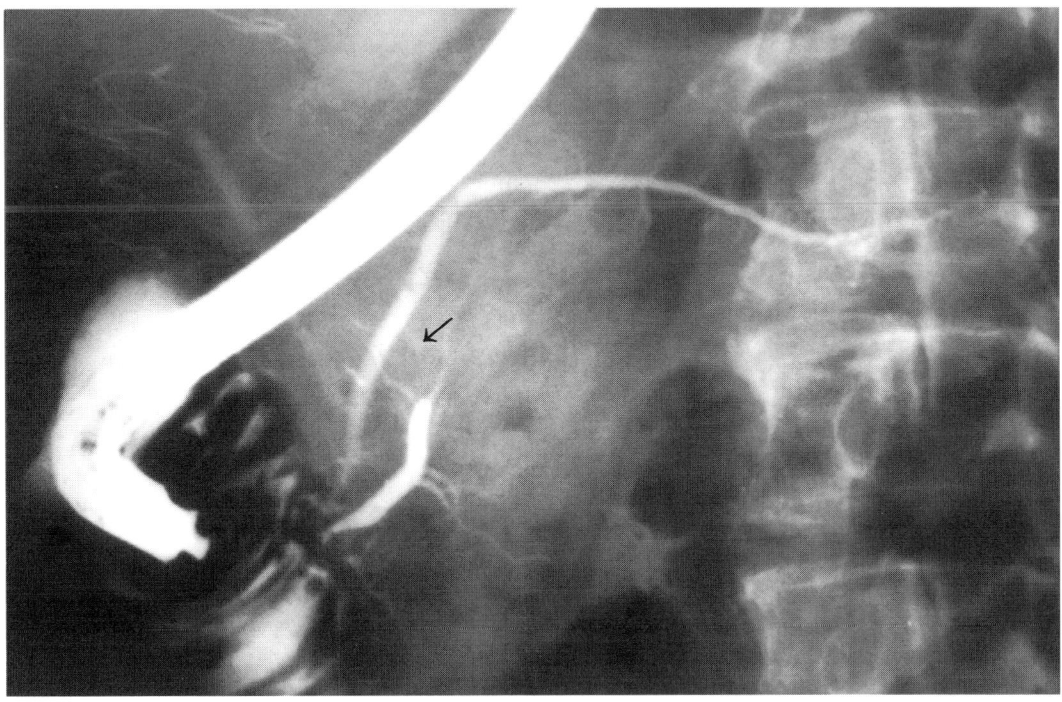

***Figure 4.21***
Incomplete pancreas divisum. Filling of the ventral duct and its branches. A communicating branch (↑) opacifies the dorsal pancreatic duct.

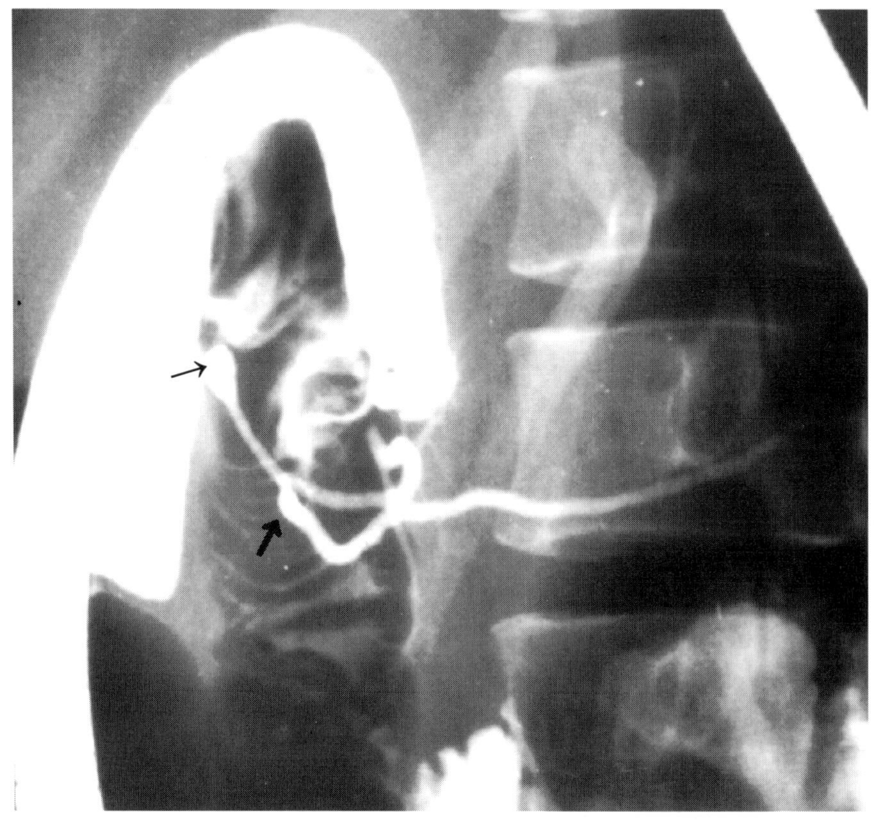

***Figure 4.22***
Incomplete pancreas divisum. Cannulation of the minor papilla. Cystic dilatation (↑) (Santorinicele) at its orifice. Filling of the dorsal pancreatic duct. A communicating branch filled the ventral duct of the pancreas (↑) and the duct of the uncinary process.

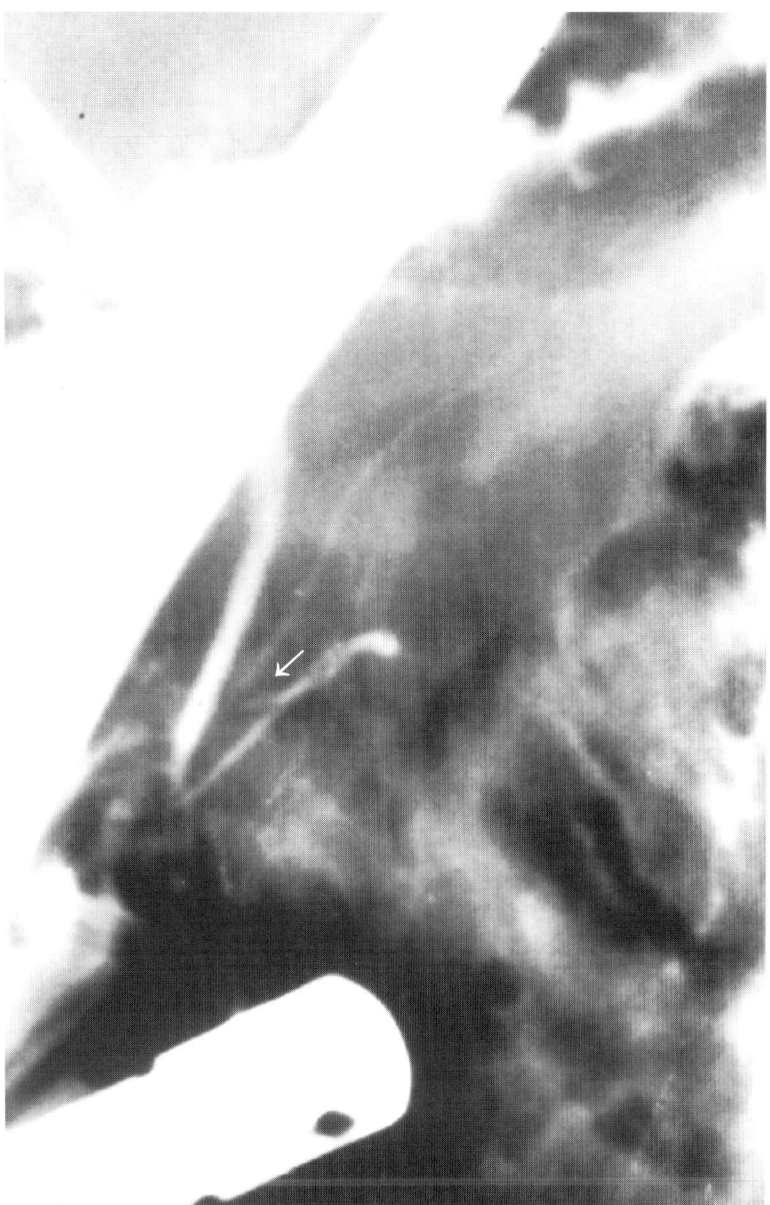

**_Figure 4.23_**

Incomplete pancreas divisum in a 2-year-old boy with recurrent pancreatitis. Filling of the ventral duct. A communicating branch (↑) opacifies a normal dorsal pancreatic duct.

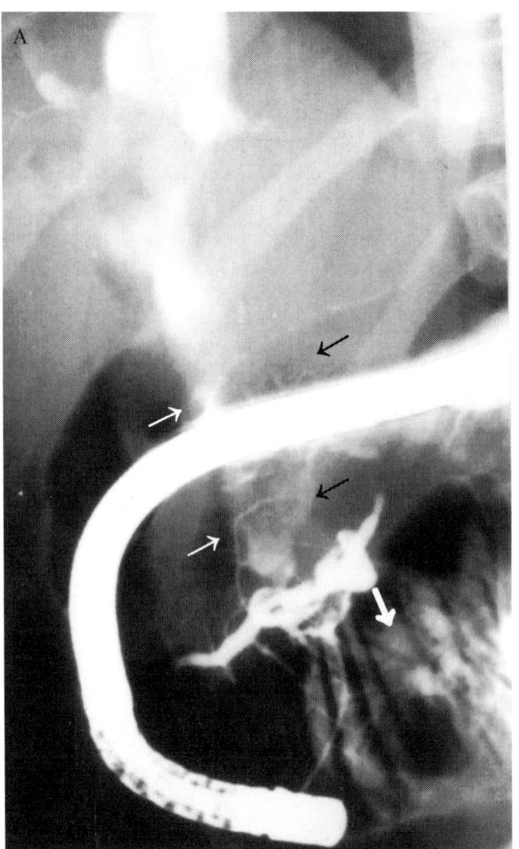
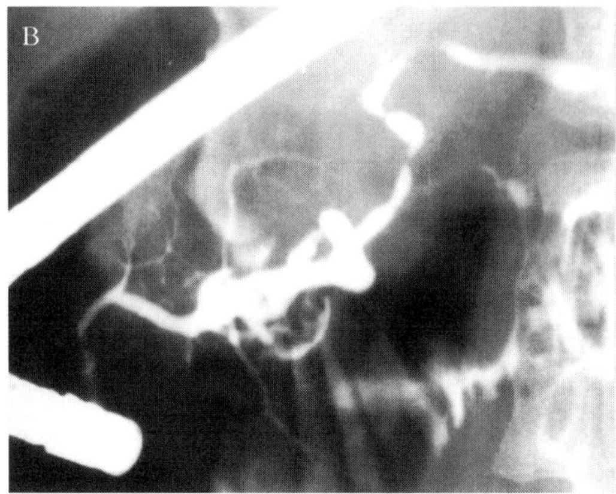

**Figure 4.24**

Incomplete pancreas divisum and choledochal cyst. (A) Cannulation of the major papilla located in the third portion of the duodenum. A choledochal cyst (type IV A) is observed (↑). A small pancreatic branch (↑) opacified the dorsal pancreatic duct which is tortuous, dilated with multiple strictures and beading of the duct. (B) Cannulation of the minor papilla located in the lower part of the second portion of the duodenum. A minor papilla sphincterotomy without stent placement was successfully performed. The patient underwent cyst resection with hepatojejunostomy and dual surgical sphincteroplasty. He remained asymptomatic for the following 2 years.

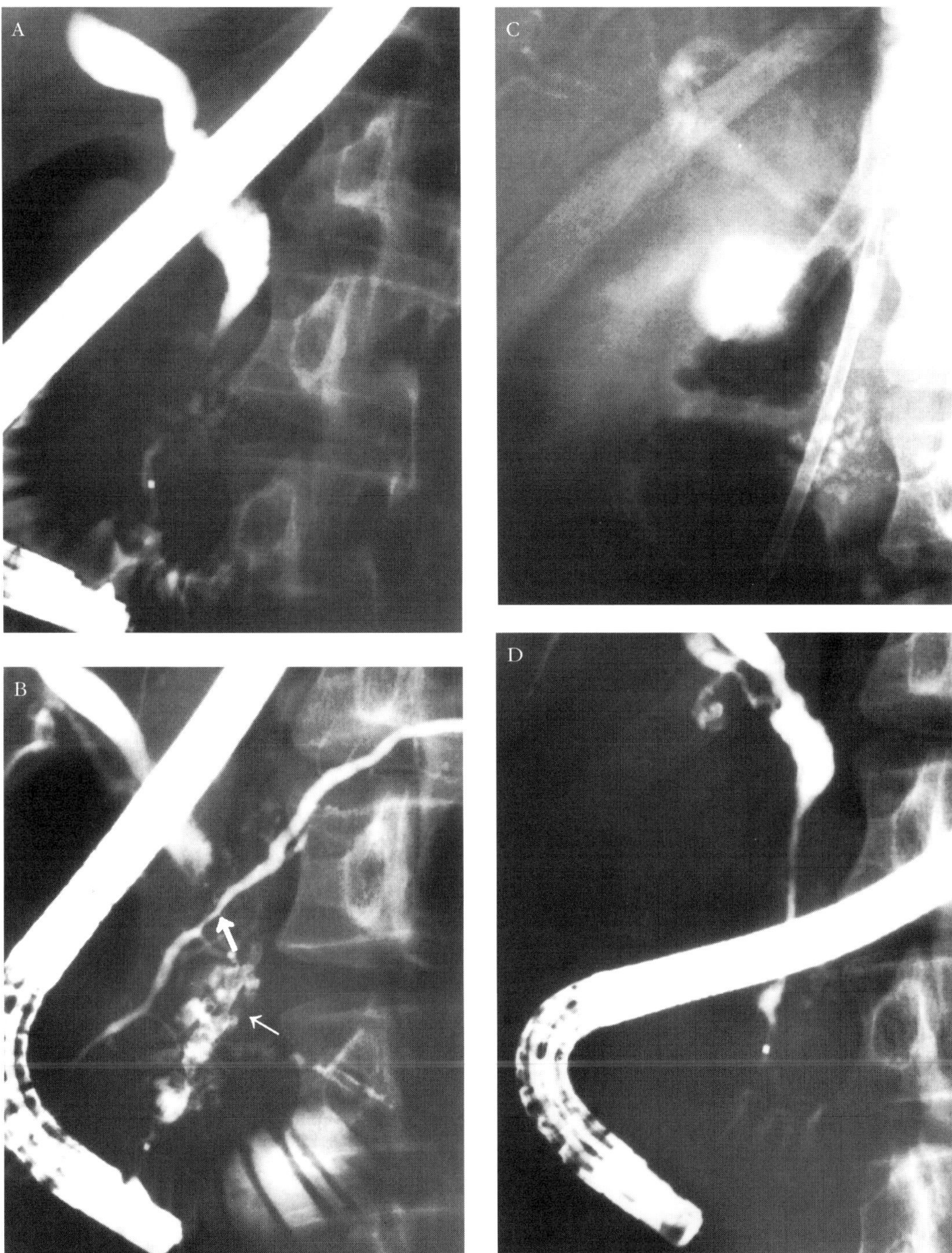

***Figure 4.25***

Incomplete pancreas divisum and chronic pancreatitis of the ventral pancreas in a jaundiced 16-year-old male. (A) A cholangiogram showing narrowing of the middle common bile duct and dilatation of the biliary tree. Multiple calcification at the head of the pancreas. (B) A pancreatogram showing severe changes of chronic pancreatitis characterized by dilated, tortuous ventral pancreatic duct (↑) with blunted, dilated secondary and tertiary branches, and multiple lucent defects in the duct. A small communicating branch (↑) filled a tortuous and dilated dorsal pancreatic duct. (C) After an endoscopic sphincterotomy of the major papilla a 10-French biliary stent is placed. (D) After 3 months follow-up, the biliary stent was extracted. A cholangiogram showed persistent common bile duct narrowing. The serum bilirubin levels were normal. After a 14-month-follow-up, the patient developed acute cholestasis. A choledochojejunostomy was performed.

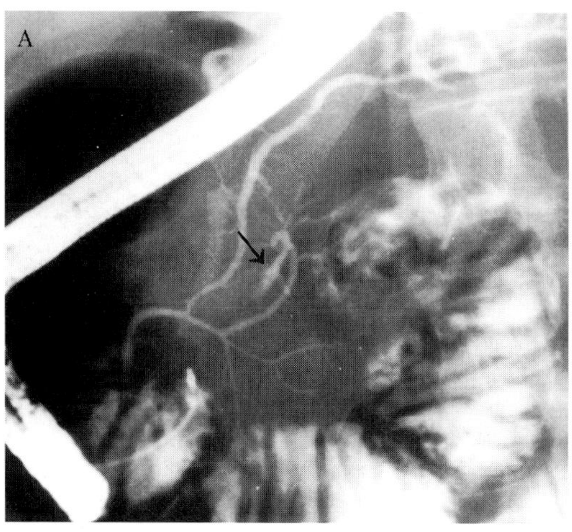
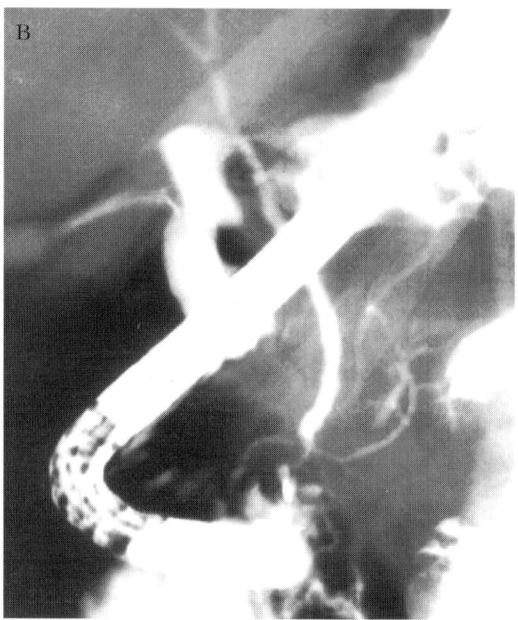

***Figure 4.26***

Incomplete pancreas divisum and isolated ventral chronic pancreatitis with sphincter of Oddi dysfunction in a 16-year-old female. (A) Cannulation of the minor papilla. Opacification of a normal dorsal duct system with normal uncinate process duct and branching of the duct. A normal caliber branch derived from the uncinate process duct opacified a dilated and tortuous ventral duct (↑) and distal branches. (B) Cannulation of the major papilla. Deformity of the distal common duct with normal common bile duct. Delayed drainage of the dorsal pancreatic duct.

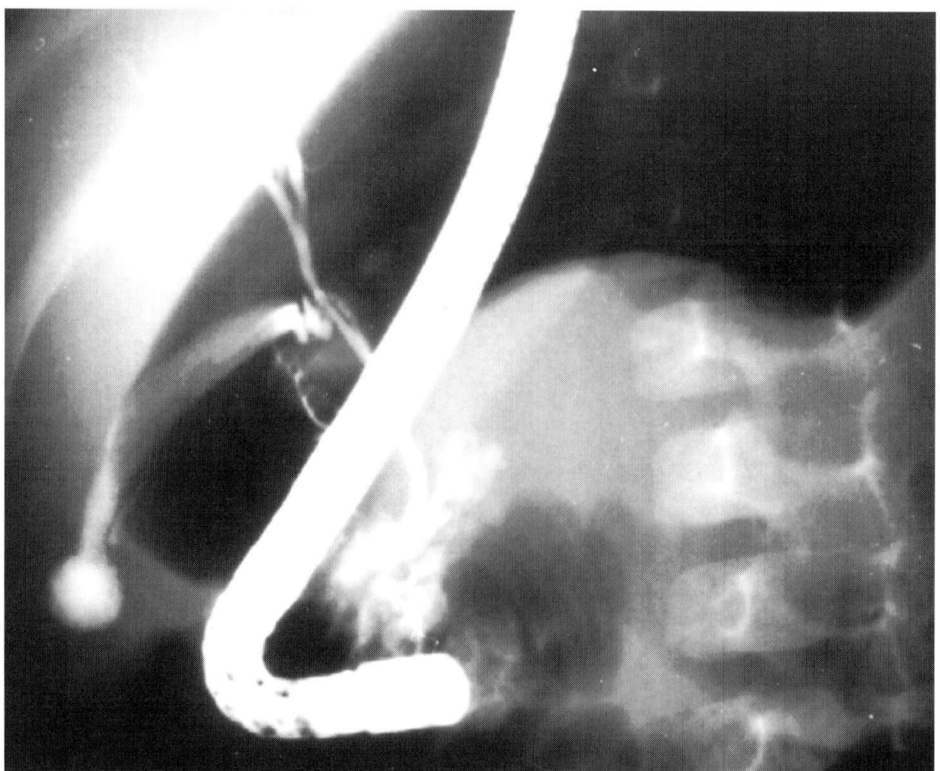

***Figure 4.27***

Pancreas divisum in a 30-day-old neonate with neonatal hepatitis. The ventral pancreas and acinogram are visualized. No attempt was made to cannulate the minor papilla.

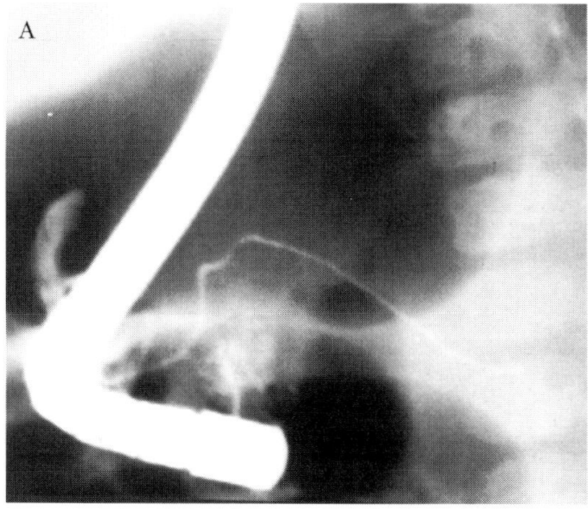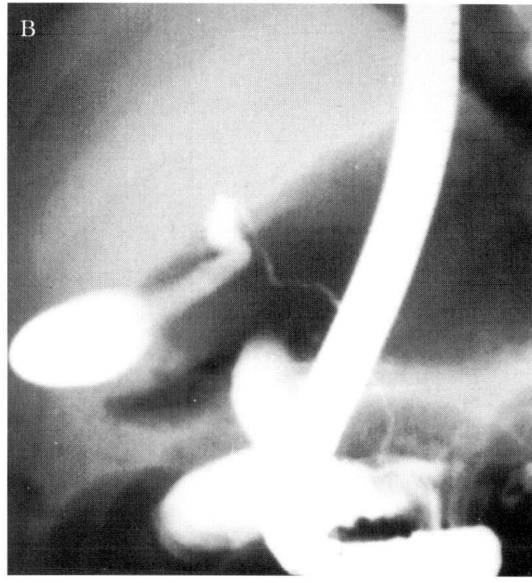

*Figure 4.28*

Pancreas divisum in a 26-day-old neonate with biliary atresia. (A) A normal appearing papilla was cannulated and only the pancreatic duct (dorsal pancreas) was visualized. (B) In an attempt to demonstrate a patent biliary tree, several maneuvers were made and the main papilla was seen 1 cm distally. Cannulation of this papilla showed a tortuous, stenotic common bile duct with visualization of the gallbladder without plenification of the intrahepatic ducts (Type 2 ERCP pattern of biliary atresia).

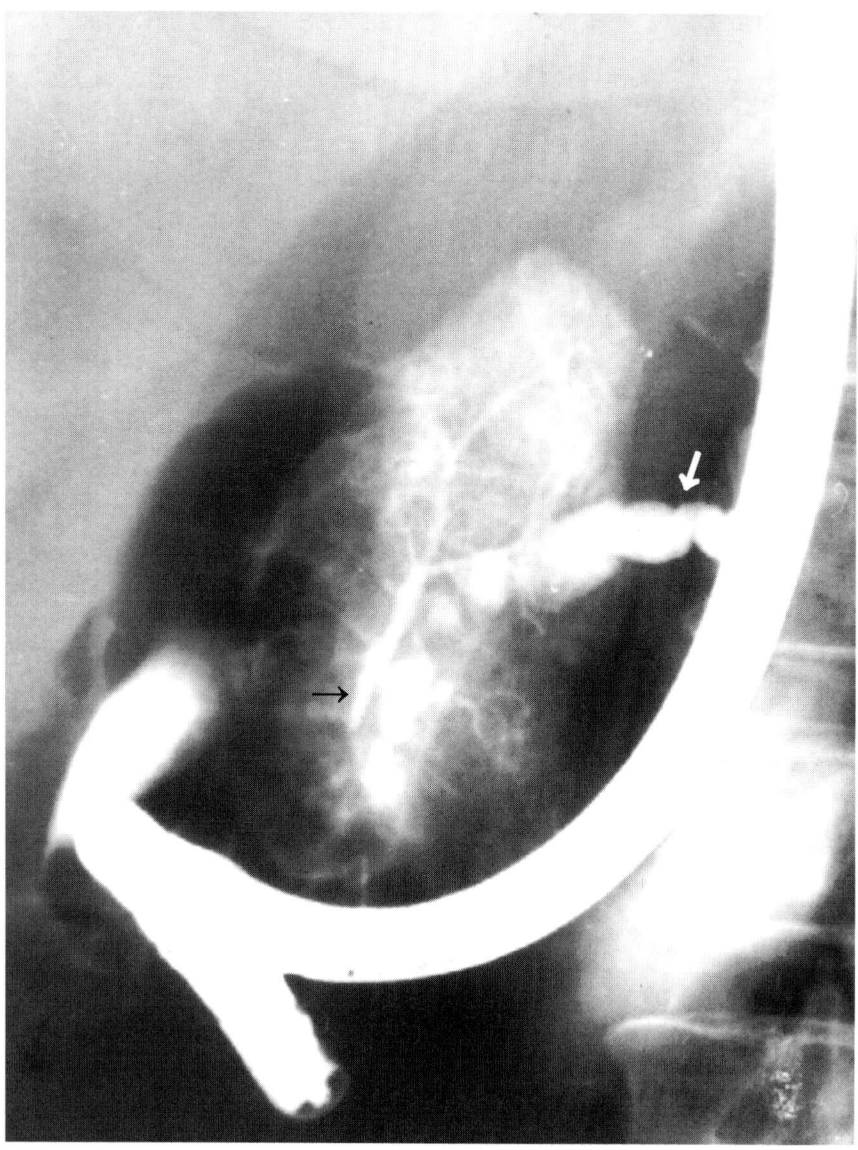

***Figure 4.29***

Pancreas divisum and chronic pancreatitis in a 12-year-old male with recurrent pancreatitis. A ventral duct (↑) with normal branches and acinogram. Separate cannulation of the minor papilla demonstrated a dilated and tortuous dorsal pancreatic duct (↑).

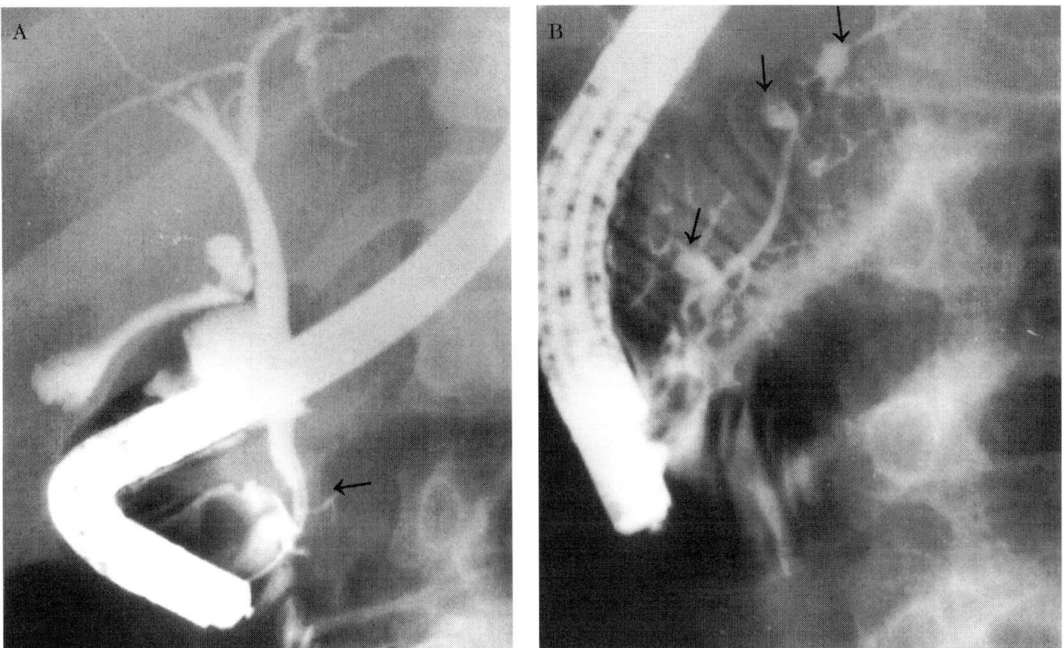

***Figure 4.30***

Pancreas divisum and pancreatic pseudocysts in a 10-year-old male after an attack of acute pancreatitis. (A) Normal biliary tree. Small ventral pancreatic duct (↑). (B) Normal appearing dorsal pancreatic duct with three small pseudocysts (↑).

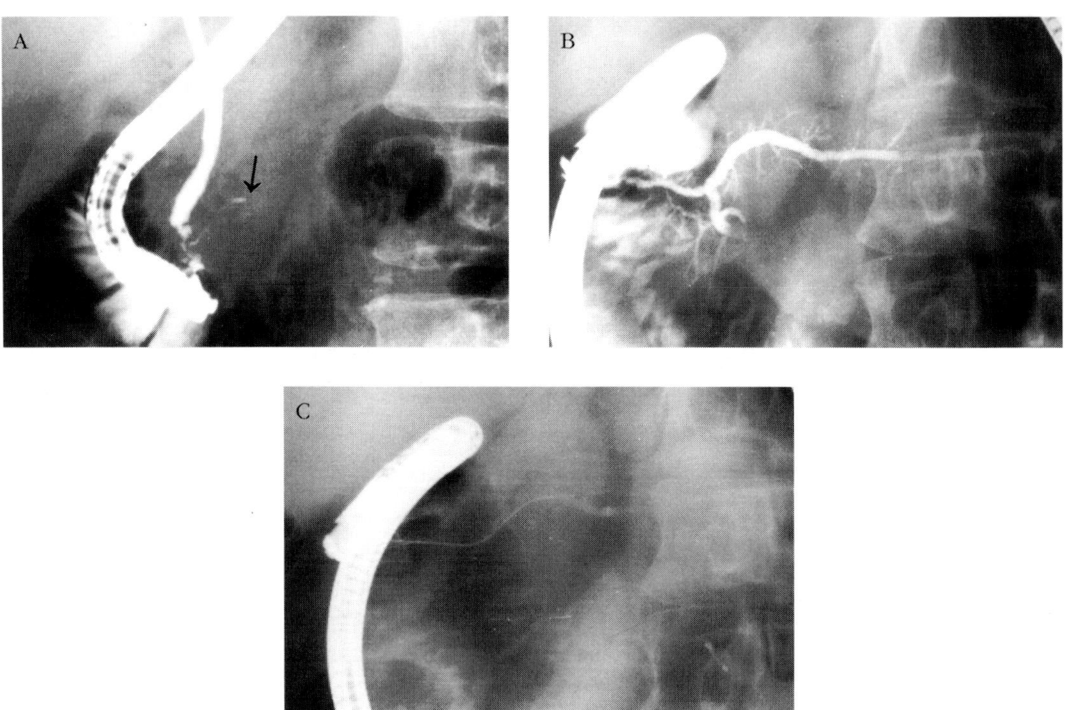

***Figure 4.31***

Pancreas divisum and chronic pancreatitis in a 17-year-old female. (A) Rudimentary ventral pancreatic duct (↑). Irregular and narrowed distal common bile duct probably due to chronic pancreatitis of the dorsal pancreas producing encasement of the bile duct. (B) Dilated dorsal pancreatic duct with dilation of primary and secondary branches. (C) A guide wire in the dorsal pancreatic duct helps in the introduction of a sphincterotome. Minor papilla sphincterotomy was performed using cutting current. No stent was left in place. In a 18-month follow-up the patient had occasional epigastric pain without pancreatic enzyme elevation.

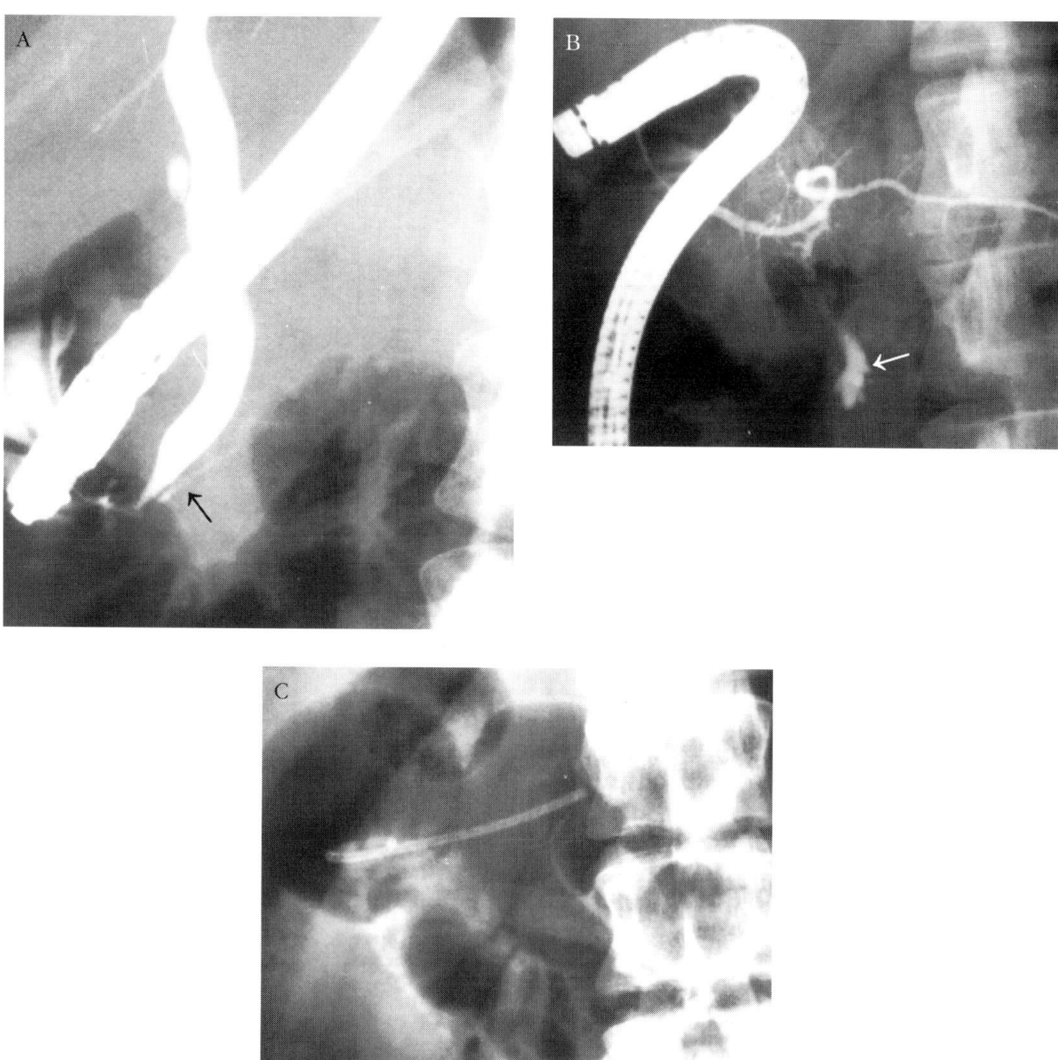

**Figure 4.32**

Pancreas divisum and pancreatic pseudocyst in a 19-year-old male. (A) Normal biliary tree. Small ventral pancreatic duct (↑). (B) Irregular and dilated dorsal pancreatic duct. Cystic cavity (↑) at the pancreatic branch of the uncinate process. (C) After minor papilla sphincterotomy, a 5-French pancreatic stent was left in place for 30 days. The patient remained asymptomatic for the following 14 months.

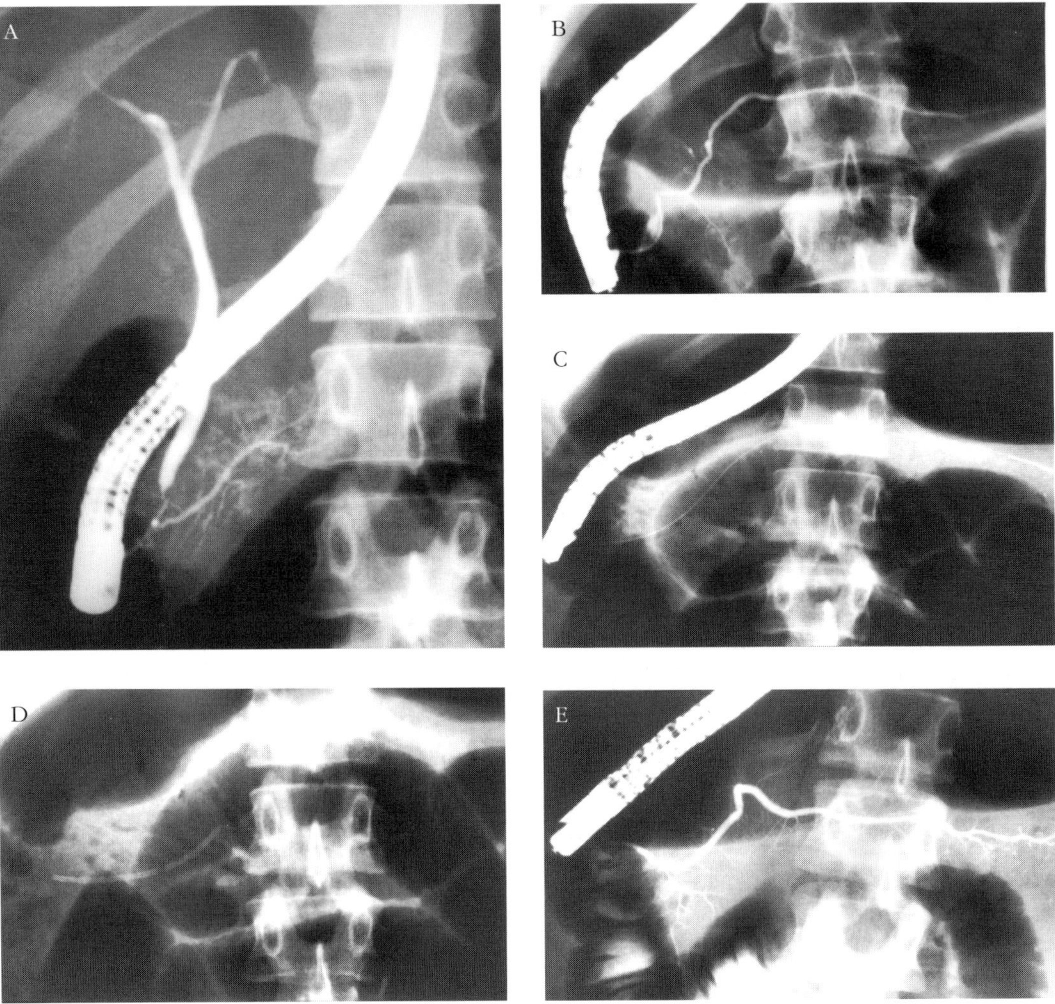

**Figure 4.33**

Pancreas divisum and endoscopic therapy in a 14-year-old female with recurrent pancreatitis. (A) Normal ventral pancreatic duct with normal branches. Normal common bile duct. (B) Normal dorsal pancreatic duct with normal uncinate process duct and branching of the duct. This configuration is unusual because the uncinate process is generally considered to be derived from the ventral endodermal primordium in the fetus (45). (C) After minor papilla sphincterotomy a 0.018 inch guidewire is advanced to the tail of the dorsal pancreatic duct. (D) A 5-French pancreatic stent is left in place for 10 days. (E) After 1-year follow-up the patient remained asymptomatic. Cannulation of the minor papilla showed a normal dorsal pancreatic duct.

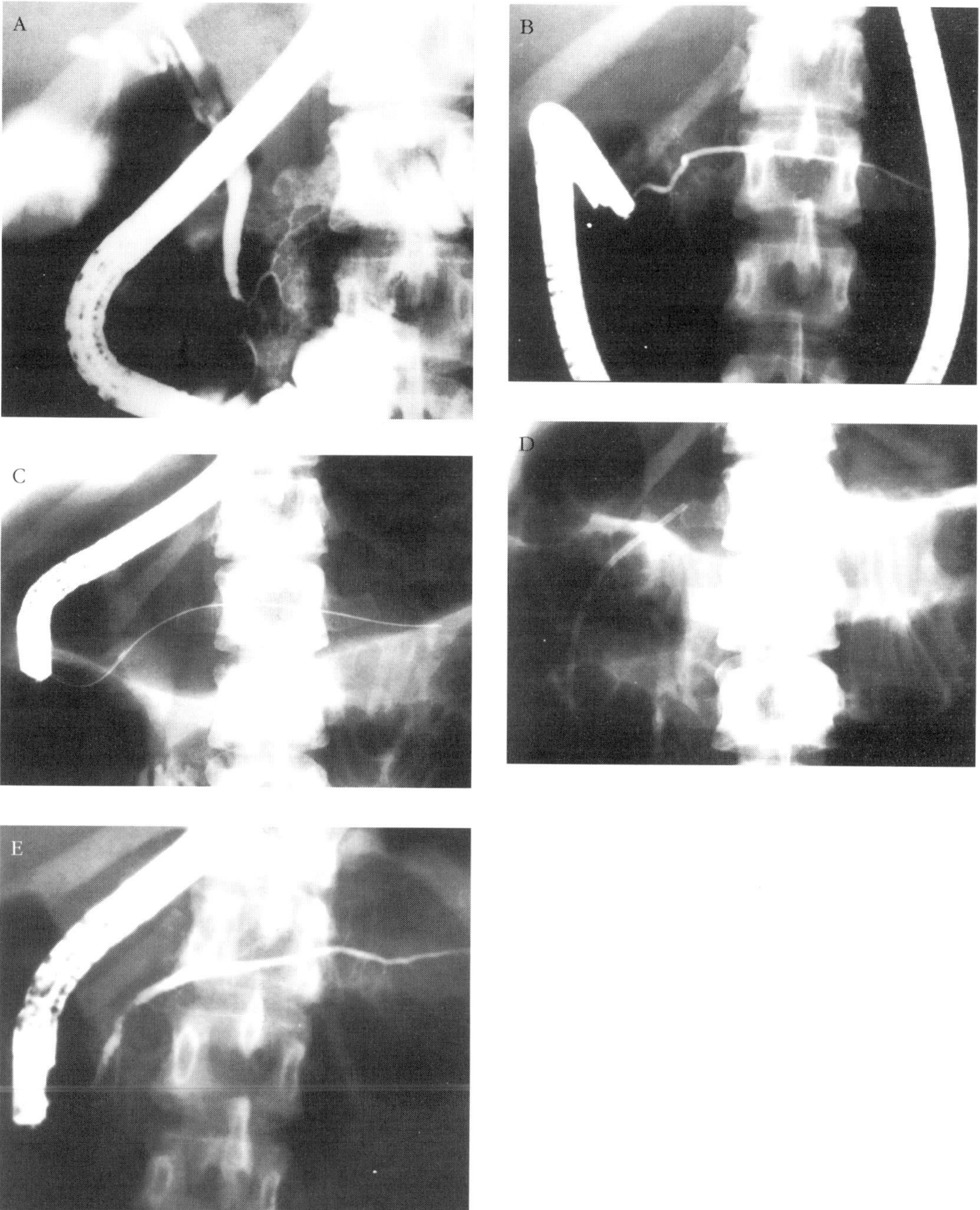

***Figure 4.34***

Pancreas divisum and dorsal pancreatic duct changes after pancreatic duct placement in a 16-year-old female with recurrent pancreatitis. (A) Normal biliary tree. Ventral pancreatic duct with normal branches and acinogram. (B) Cannulation of the minor papilla. Normal dorsal pancreatic duct. (C) Guide wire within the dorsal pancreatic duct. (D) After minor papilla sphincterotomy a 5-French pancreatic stent is left in place during 30 days. (E) After pancreatic stent retrieval, the pancreatic duct is dilated with a narrow segment where the tip of the stent was located.

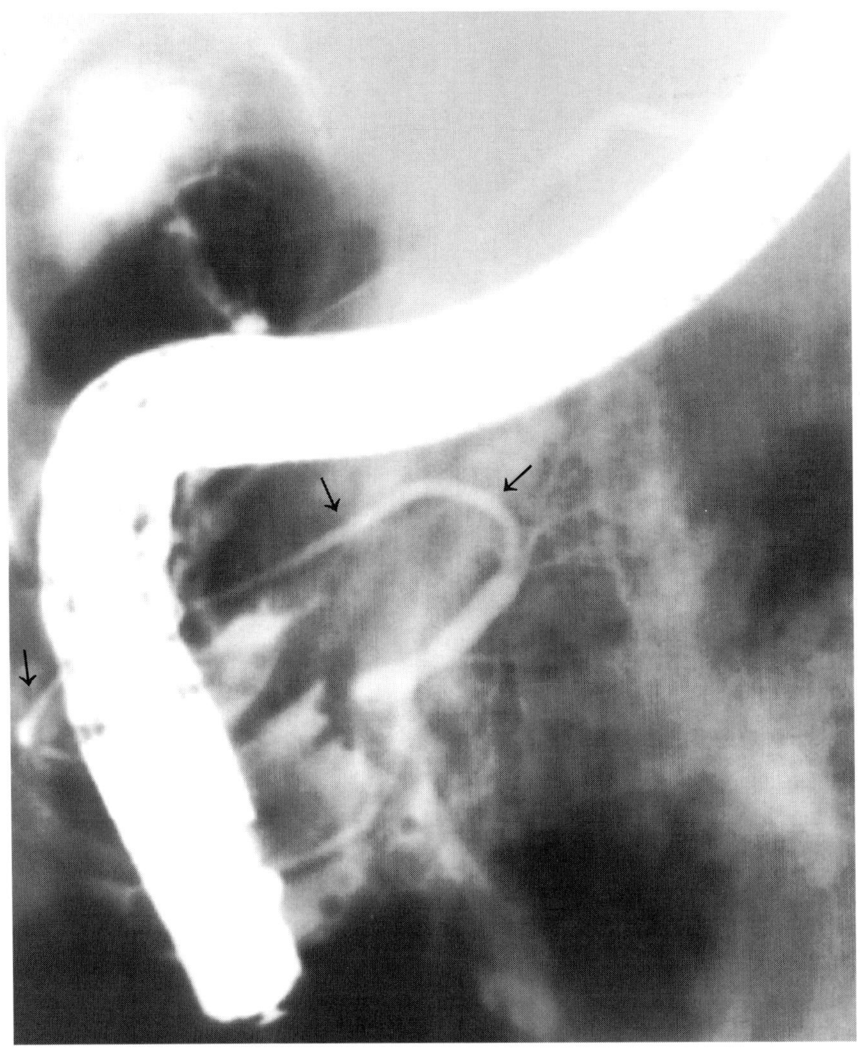

***Figure 4.35***
Annular pancreas and pancreas divisum in a 14-year-old female with recurrent pancreatitis. Cannulation of the major papilla. Short ventral pancreas with normal primary and secondary branches. A normal pancreatic duct encircles the second portion of the duodenum (↑).

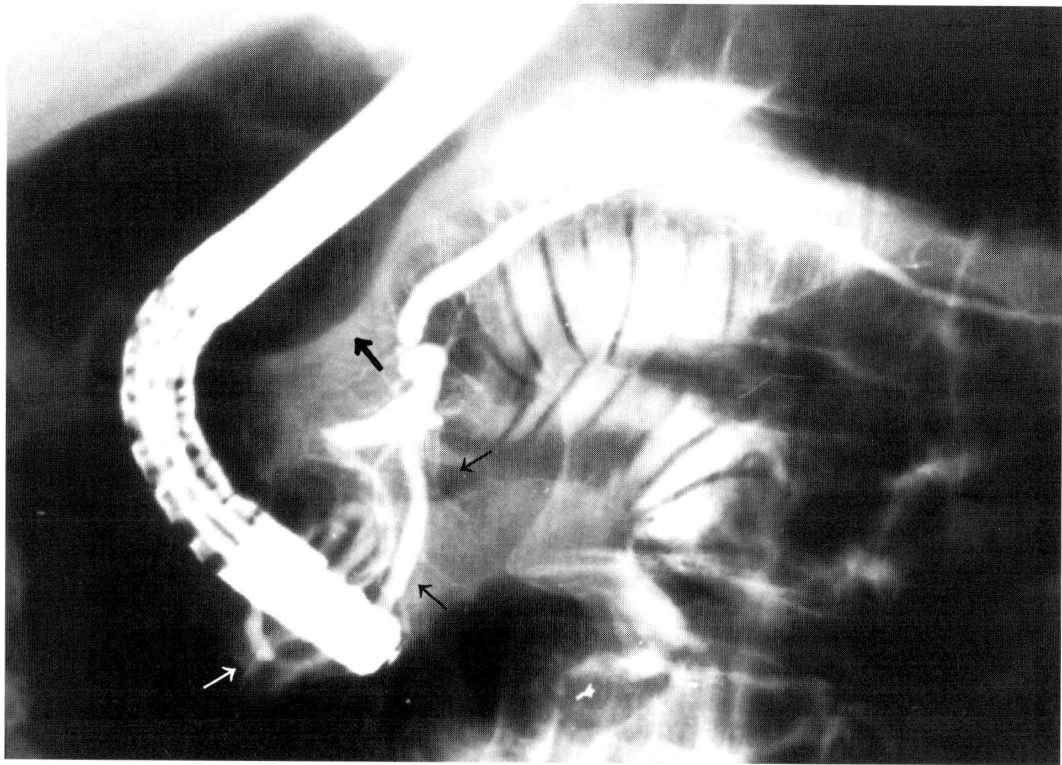

**Figure 4.36**
Annular pancreas in a 16-year-old male with recurrent pancreatitis. The pancreatic duct is dilated with a stricture (↑) at the body of the pancreas. A dilated pancreatic branch (↑) encircles the second portion of the duodenum.

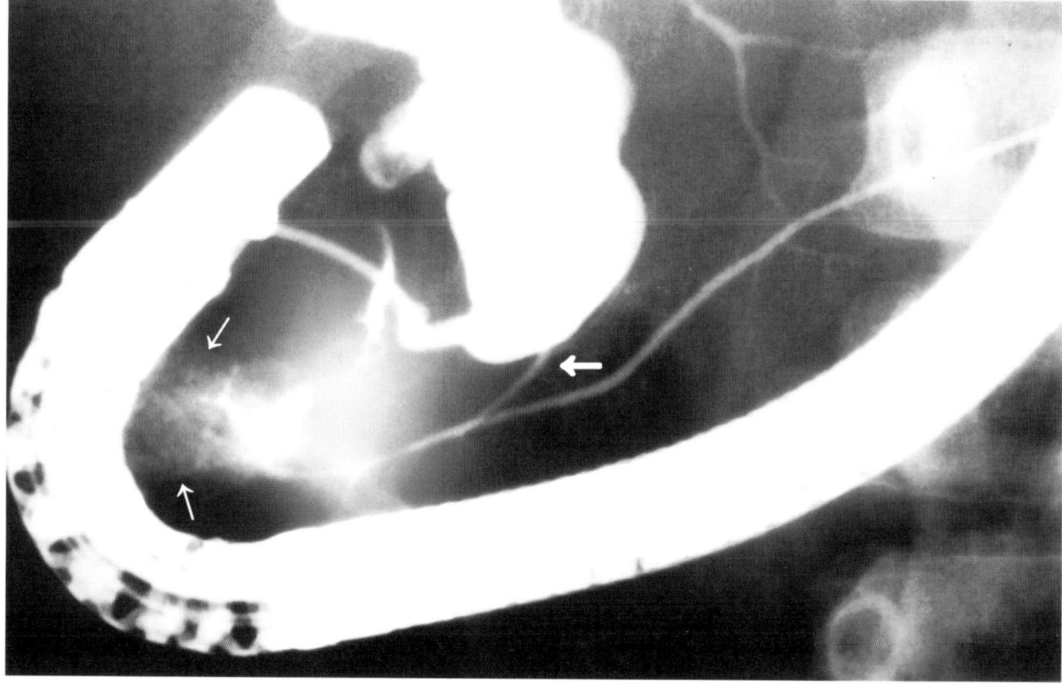

**Figure 4.37**
Annular pancreas and choledochal cyst in a 3-year-old female with recurrent pancreatitis. Anomalous pancreaticobiliary union. Type IC choledochal cyst. Normal intrahepatic ducts. Communicating pancreatic branch (↑) filled the main pancreatic duct. Acinogram (↑) in the lateral margin of the second portion of the duodenum below the main papilla.

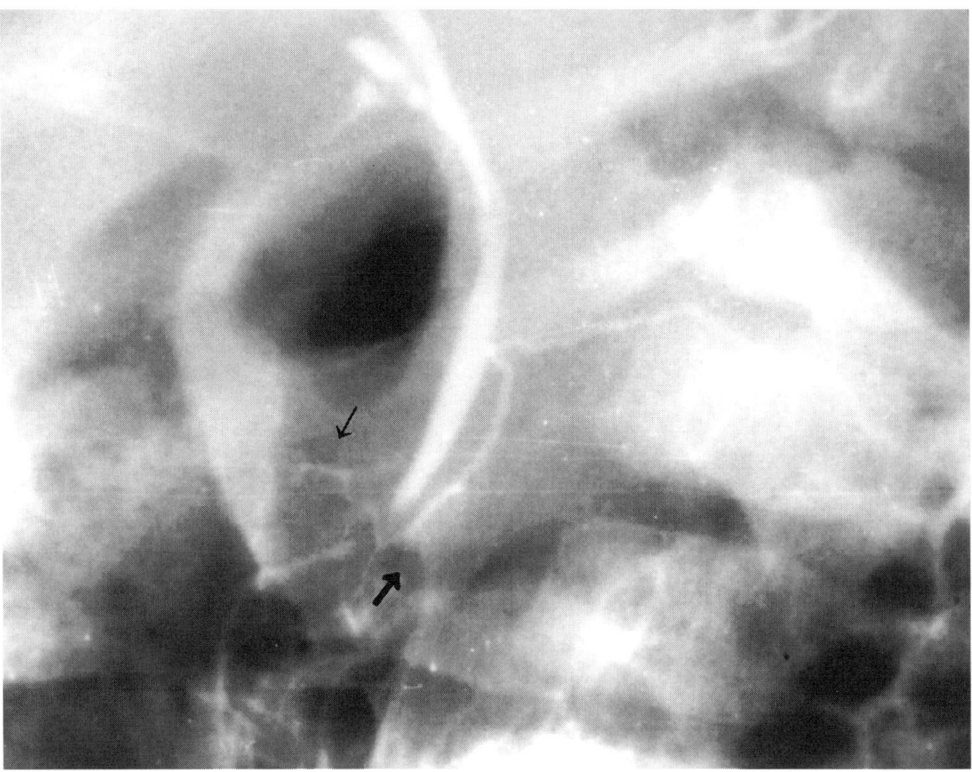

***Figure 4.38***

Annular pancreas and anomalous pancreaticobiliary union in a 18-month-old female with two attacks of acute pancreatitis in the last 3 months. Anomalous pancreaticobiliary union (↑) BP type. Normal biliary tree. Irregular pancreatic branch (↑) encircling the second portion of the duodenum.

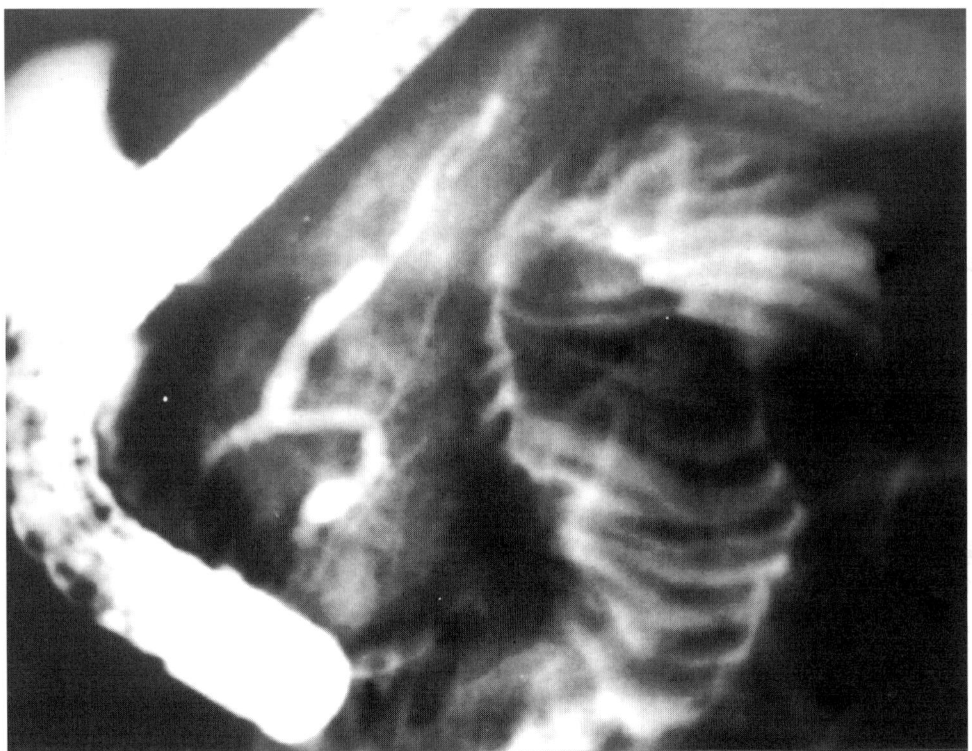

***Figure 4.39***

Short pancreas in a 3-year-old girl with recurrent pancreatitis. The main pancreatic duct and the accessory duct are dilated.

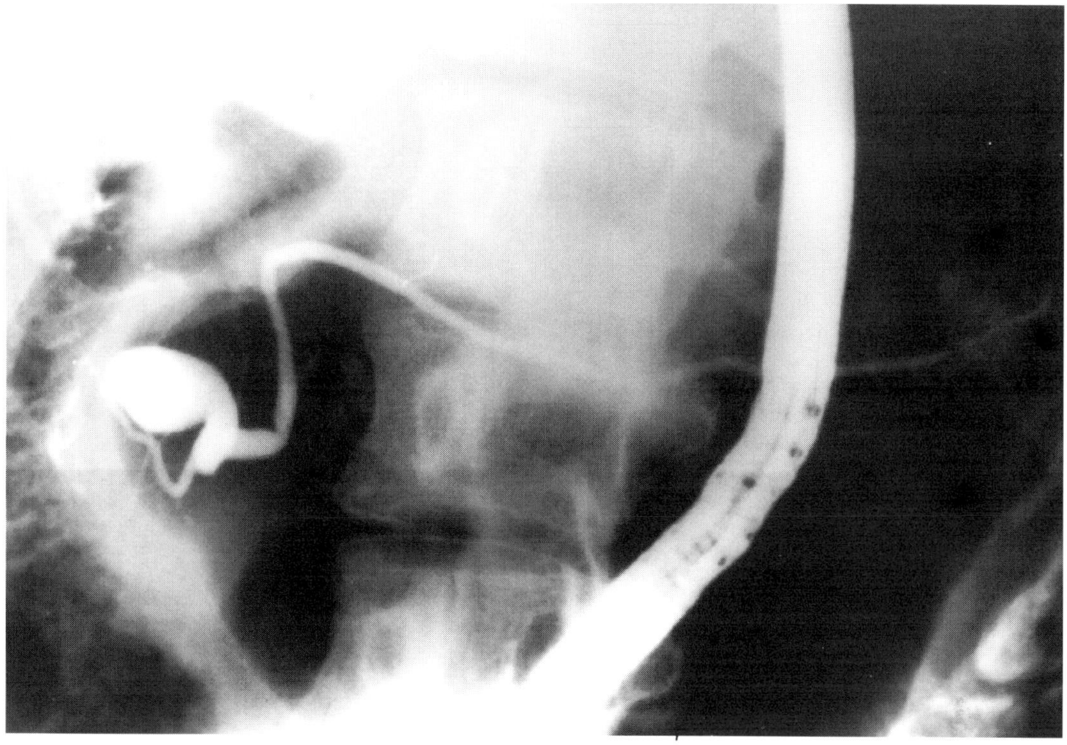

***Figure 4.40***
Cystic dilatation of the pancreatic duct (Pancreatocele) in a 14-year-old female with recurrent pancreatitis.

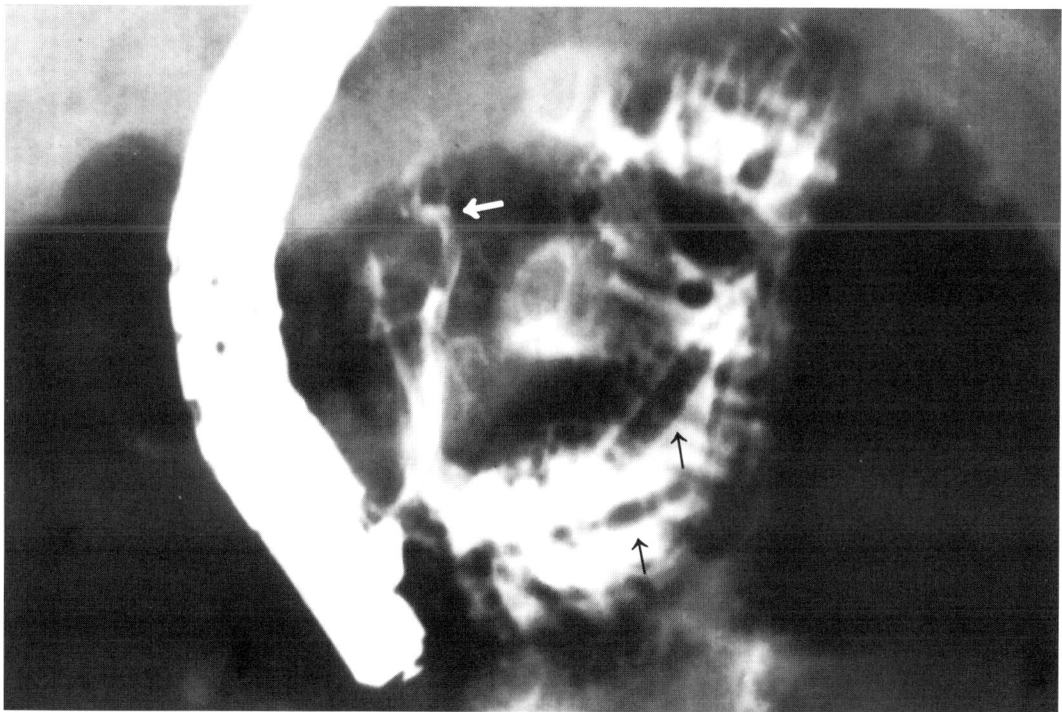

***Figure 4.41***
*Ascaris* in the pancreatic duct in a 5-year-old male with acute pancreatitis. A linear defect (↑) within the pancreatic duct is demonstrated. The worm is removed with a tripod device. Several worms are seen in the duodenum (↑).

# CHAPTER 5

# Chronic pancreatitis

Chronic pancreatitis is a progressive and insidious inflammatory disease of the pancreas that is characterized by the destruction of both exocrine and endocrine elements of the gland. Chronic pancreatitis is relatively uncommon in children, with two major morphologic pat-terns recognized: (i) chronic calcifying pancreatitis and (ii) chronic obstructive pancreatitis. The first form is marked by severe ductal epithelial damage, acinar atrophy and frequent calculi. This form in children is most often due to juvenile tropical pancreatitis or hereditary pancreatitis. The second form appears to be less common; it results in less severe damage, and stones are unusual. This form is associated with congenital or acquired lesions of the pancreatic duct, or biliary tree similar to those etiologic factors in recurrent pancreatitis. Distinction between recurrent acute pancreatitis and chronic pancreatitis is difficult as there is a continuum of gross and pathologic changes. This may not be possible early in the course of the disease, when the initial episode of chronic pancreatitis is usually interpreted as acute pancreatitis.

The predominant clinical feature is pain, which occurs in most children. Weight loss and failure to grow are also very common. Both exocrine and endocrine insufficiencies occur, with progressive destruction of the gland; diabetes and malabsorption with steatorrhea eventually develop in about half of the children (1). Little information is available concerning the natural history of chronic pancreatitis in children. Pain sometimes resolves spontaneously, but the incidence of such resolution is not known. Frequently the reduction in pain is due to complete fibrosis and atrophy of the pancreas. A few patients with chronic pancreatitis manifest pancreatic atrophy or malabsorption with no history of pain. Complications of chronic pancreatitis include jaundice due to extrahepatic bile duct obstruction, bowel obstruction, pseudocysts, pancreatic ascites, and splenic, portal or mesenteric venous thrombosis.

ERCP is the most useful imaging modality in the diagnosis of chronic pancreatitis. ERCP has been found useful in the identification of chronic pancreatitis in 14–69% of children (Table 5.1).

The earliest changes involve the side branches of the main pancreatic duct and include dilatation, contour irregularity, clubbing, stenosis of the side branches at their junction with the main pancreatic duct, and opacification of small cavities. These changes may be accompanied by mild dilatation of the main pancreatic duct (Figs 5.1 and 5.2). As the disease progresses, the involvement of the main pancreatic duct increases, producing more marked dilatation, loss of normal tapering, irregularity of the walls, areas of stenosis or occlusion of the main pancreatic duct. (Fig. 5.3). Advanced changes of chronic pancreatitis include more marked dilatation and irregularity of the main pancreatic duct with intraluminal calculi and single or multiple stenosis. Occasionally a pseudocyst may be opacified. The changes in the side branches are also more marked lesions (Figs 5.4 and 5.5). The display of ductal anatomy by ERCP is also helpful in planning the therapeutic approach to these patients.

**Table 5.1** Frequency of chronic pancreatitis in ERCP in childhood

| Author, year (reference) | No. of patients | No. of chronic pancreatitis |
|---|---|---|
| Forbes, 1984 (2) | 25 | 14 (56%) |
| Buckley, 1990 (3) | 18 | 5 (28%) |
| Putnam, 1991 (4) | 12 | 6 (50%) |
| Dite, 1992 (5) | 16 | 11 (69%) |
| Brown, 1994 (6) | 9 | 4 (44%) |
| Lemmel, 1994 (7) | 29 | 6 (21%) |
| Guelrud, 1994 (8) | 50 | 7 (14%) |
| Total | 159 | 53 (33%) |

## Juvenile tropical pancreatitis

This is the most common form of chronic pancreatitis in children (1). The disease is characterized by chronic abdominal pain, diabetes mellitus and pancreatic calculi. The disease appears to be associated with protein malnutrition. The term malnutrition indicates a wide spectrum of nutritional disorders that collectively serve to accelerate or precipitate pancreatic disease. Dietary toxins (Cassava root) and micronutrient deficiencies are considered to be coexisting, also unproved as casual factors (9). The symptoms and physical examination are non-specific. The diagnosis is suggested by the association of diabetes mellitus and chronic abdominal pain. Abdominal ultrasound and CT demonstrate pancreatic calcifications.

ERCP demonstrates evidence of ductular dilatation or obstruction with calculi (Fig. 5.6). Frequently, surgical therapy is complicated by the nutritional status of the patient (10). In these cases, endoscopic sphincterotomy of the pancreatic sphincter with stone extraction (Fig. 5.7) constitutes an excellent alternative to relieve recurrent abdominal pain and to avoid progressive parenchymal damage to the pancreas (8,11).

## Hereditary pancreatitis

This is an autosomal dominant disorder characterized by recurrent attacks of mild to moderate pancreatitis. Pancreatic insufficiency and diabetes mellitus may occur in half of the patients. The diagnosis is obvious when another member of the family has idiopathic recurrent pancreatitis. ERCP may demonstrate dilatation of the main duct with large, rounded intraductal calcifying stones. In cases with severe recurrent pain or relapsing episodes of pancreatitis, endoscopic sphincterotomy with stone extraction (Fig. 5.8) may improve the outcome of these patients (8,11). However, these patients frequently require more than one procedure for palliation of pain, including surgery, and overall results have been disappointing in many instances (1).

## Idiopathic fibrosing pancreatitis

This is a rare form of chronic pancreatitis in children (12,13). The disease is characterized by painless obstructive jaundice. Intermittent, non-specific pain syndromes have been described, but many patients are entirely pain-free. Clinical evidence of chronic pancreatitis is generally lacking, with calcification in the pancreas unusual. The diagnosis requires the exclusion of other etiologies. Ultrasound reveals a dilated biliary tree and, less often, an enlarged pancreas. ERCP shows a dilated common bile duct with distal narrowing at the level of the pancreas. The main pancreatic duct is frequently abnormal (14,15). ERCP provides the most definitive information about the common bile duct and the pancreatic duct, before endoscopic or surgical therapy. ERCP findings may masquerade as a "double-duct" sign of pancreatic carcinoma in adults but this is very rare in children (Fig. 5.13).

## Therapy

Therapeutic ERCP has been rarely applied as a tool for the treatment of chronic pancreatitis in children (8,11). In children with chronic pancreatitis, recurrent attacks may be caused by strictures of the main duct, pancreatic stones or pseudocysts that impair the normal outflow of pancreatic juice. Most successful treatment of pain in chronic pancreatitis has been based on the concept of pancreatic duct decompression (16) (Table 5.2).

***Table 5.2*** Endoscopic therapy for recurrent or chronic pancreatitis

| Clinical condition | Endoscopic therapy |
| --- | --- |
| Recurrent or chronic pancreatitis | Endoscopic sphincterotomy of the bile duct and/or pancreatic duct<br>Stricture dilation<br>Stone extraction (ESWL, mechanical or electrohydraulic lithotriptor, laser)<br>Bile duct and/or pancreatic duct stents<br>Pancreatic duct occlusion (histoacryl) |
| Pseudocyst, duct disruption, ascites | Cystoenterostomy<br>Transpapillary drainage |
| Pancreas divisum | Minor papilla sphincterotomy<br>Dorsal pancreatic stent |

In adults, strictures of the main duct are endoscopically treated by endoscopic stent placement across the stricture. Endoprostheses have been used in a short term to select patients who might be expected to respond to decompression surgery. The results have been equivocal (17). Typically, endoprostheses have been used long-term, with or without concomitant dilation (18–21). Placement of such stents is possible in about 85% of patients in which it is attempted. Most patients obtain temporary pain relief (90%). Sustained pain relief of up to 69 months after stent removal has been observed (20). The length of time stents were left within the pancreatic duct varied from weeks to several months. Recently, Guelrud *et al.* performed a dual endoscopic sphincterotomy of the pancreatic duct and common duct followed by a pancreatic stent placement during 2 weeks in three children with dilated pancreatic duct chronic pancreatitis and debilitating pancreatic pain. Two patients experienced significant improvement during a 2-year follow-up period (8).

Aggravation or development of duct changes mimicking chronic pancreatitis may develop during the stent treatment (22–24). Because of the stent induced lesions, we are reluctant to recommend long-term stenting in children.

Pancreatic duct stones can be treated by endoscopic sphincterotomy of the pancreatic duct followed by extraction of the stone (Figs 5.7–5.10) (25–28). Kozarek *et al.* (11) performed pancreatic duct sphincterotomy followed by stone extraction and stent insertion in three children with chronic relapsing pancreatitis, after which marked improvement in chronic abdominal pain was noted. Brown *et al.* (29) performed pancreatic and biliary sphincterotomy followed by balloon dilation of a mid-pancreatic duct stricture and by pancreatic stone removal in a 2-year-old child with hereditary pancreatitis with excellent results in a 10-month follow-up.

Endoscopic extraction of pancreatic calculi may be impossible due to large stones, or stones located behind ductal strictures, or stones adherent to the ductal wall. These calculi can be fragmented with mechanical, electrohydraulic, extracorporeal shock-wave lithotripsy or laser lithotripsy (30–33). There is no experience in children with these techniques.

Endoscopic occlusion of the pancreatic duct has been proposed as a treatment for patients with chronic pancreatitis and intractable pain (34). The idea was that permanent occlusion of the pancreatic ducts leads to atrophy of the exocrine parenchyma and fibrotic transformation, without primary damage to the islets cells. Burning the exocrine pancreas would offer no substrate for further attacks of pancreatitis. This technique has been abandoned by Rosch (35) who noted poor long-term results. Although most of his patients had an intact pancreas, apparently the instillation pressure via an endoscopic cannula is not strong enough to guarantee complete filling of the main pancreatic duct and the primary and secondary branches. Guelrud *et al.* performed occlusion of the pancreatic duct with cyanoacrilate glue in a narcotic addicted adolescent female with chronic pancreatitis and intractable pain (Fig. 5.11). A previous subtotal pancreatectomy allowed for complete filling of the ductal system. Freedom from pain was achieved for 2 years. After a second cyanoacrilate injection was performed, she remained symptom-free for 3 years (8).

The short-term symptomatic relief reported in 4 series (6–7,11) probably relates to ductal decompression (Table 5.3). Whether symptom relief will be sustained remains conjectural because the longest follow-up to date in these children is 3 years (8). Endoscopic therapy may provide palliation and allow growth and development to occur before the need for surgical decompressive procedure. When performed by experienced endoscopists, therapeutic pancreatography can be successfully performed in a selected group of children with a low rate of complications. A longer follow-up period will be necessary to determine whether presumed successful endoscopic therapy produces long-standing clinical improvement.

**Table 5.3.** Symptomatic improvement after pancreatic endoscopic therapy in children

| Author, year (reference) | No. of patients treated | Improved |
| --- | --- | --- |
| Kozarek, 1993 (11) | 5 | 4 (80%) |
| Brown, 1994 (6) | 6 | 6 (100%) |
| Lemmel, 1994 (7) | 9 | 6 (67%) |
| Guelrud, 1994 (8) | 18 | 15 (83%) |
| Total | 38 | 31 (82%) |

## Pseudocysts

Pancreatic pseudocysts are a common consequence of acute and chronic pancreatitis (10–50%) (36–38). They are well defined, rounded fluid masses situated either outside or within the limits of the pancreas. In chronic pancreatitis most pseudocysts are presumably produced by increased intraductal pressure leading to rupture of a duct with leakage of pancreatic fluid that is demarcated from surrounding structures by a capsule composed of inflammatory reaction. Pseudocysts can also complicate an acute attack of pancreatitis with extravasation of enzyme rich fluid through damaged pancreatic ducts. A fibrous capsule of inflammatory reaction and fibrosis encircles the fluid forming a round mass. Pancreatic pseudocysts resolve spontaneously in up to 85% of acute pancreatitis (39) and in 9% of patients with chronic pancreatitis (40)). Symptomatic, large ( >4 cm), or persistent pseudocysts beyond 6 weeks are unlikely to resolve and are at risk of severe complications (41). In these cases treatment is indicated.

There has been increased interest in non-operative management of pancreatic pseudocysts. The success of treatment by percutaneous aspiration or drainage catheter placement has been variable. Pseudocysts recur in 10–15% of percutaneously drained fluid collections (42). Pseudocysts which communicate with the pancreatic ductal system are particularly refractory to percutaneous techniques.

In the last 15 years, endoscopic methods have developed as an alternative to surgical treatment and percutaneous drainage of pancreatic pseudocysts. These endoscopic methods include endoscopic cystogastrostomy, cystoduodenostomy, and transpapillary drainage. Candidates for endoscopic cystogastrostomy or cystoduodenostomy are patients with a pseudocyst greater than 4 cm which obviously bulges into the duodenal or gastric lumen. The cyst wall should be mature and the distance from lumen to cyst cavity should be < 1 cm by ultrasound or CT. A needle knife is used to cut a hole into the cyst cavity. The cyst cavity is penetrated with a catheter and a wire guided stent is left for drainage. The communication may be expanded with a sphincterotome or needle knife. When compared to other endoscopic techniques, this technique has a relatively high bleeding and perforation rate. Nevertheless, the overall complication rate probably compares favorably to surgical series. Cremer *et al.* reported their results in 33 patients including 22 in whom they performed a cystoduodenostomy and 11 in whom a cystogastrostomy was performed (43). Technical success rates were 96% and 100% respectively with successful pseudocyst resolution in 82% of the cases. Similar results have been reported by others (44–46).

Transpapillary drainage offers another approach to pseudocyst management, and is applicable to pseudocysts of the head and body which communicate with the main duct. If a guide wire can be manipulated into the pseudocyst *per se*, a stent can be placed into the pseudocyst with or without the help of pancreatic sphincterotomy. Huibregtse *et al.* reported transpapillary pseudocyst drainage in six patients, five of whom had excellent results (20). Kozarek *et al.* placed transpapillary drains in 17 patients with pancreatic duct disruption, nine with acute and eight with chronic pancreatitis, with excellent results in 14 patients (47). Barthet *et al.* treated 30 patients with pancreatic pseudocysts with ductal communication by endoscopic transpapillary cyst drainage (22 patients) and by cystenterostomies (10 patients) (48). Twenty-six (87%) patients had pseudocyst resolution, but three ultimately required surgery for early recurrence. Catalano *et al.* treated 21 patients with pancreatic pseudocysts with ductal communication by transpapillary pancreatic duct endoprosthesis (49). Initial resolution of pseudocysts was seen in 17 patients, with 16 patients (76%) free of pseudocyst recurrence at mean follow-up of 37 months. Binmoeller *et al.* performed transpapillary drainage of pancreatic pseudocysts (50). Endoscopic drainage was technically successful in 50 patients (94%), of whom 47 had complete pseudocyst resolution. Mean follow-up was 22 months; pseudocysts recurred in 11 patients (23%), of whom seven were successfully re-treated endoscopically. Surgery can be reserved for those patients in whom endoscopic therapy fails. Such maneuvers were performed in three of our children with non-resolving communicating pseudocysts (8). In one child the procedure was unsuccessful for technical reasons. Two children became asymptomatic after transampullary endoprosthesis placement (Fig. 5.12). The pseudocysts resolved rapidly. After follow-up of 2 and 3 years, both patients remained asymptomatic without pseudocysts demonstrated on ultrasound.

# References

1. Piccoli D. Chronic pancreatitis. In Wyllie R, Hyams JS, eds: *Pediatric Gastrointestinal Disease. Pathophysiology, Diagnosis and Management.* Philadelphia: W. B. Saunders Company, 1993: 880–92.

2. Forbes A, Leung JWC, Cotton PB. Relapsing acute and chronic pancreatitis. *Arch Dis Child* 1984; **59:** 927–34.

3. Buckley A, Connon JJ. The role of ERCP in children and adolescents. *Gastrointest Endosc* 1990; **36:** 369–72.

4. Putnam PE, Kocoshis SA, Orenstein SR, Schade RR. Pediatric endoscopic retrograde cholangiopancreatography. *Am J Gastroenterol* 1991; **86:** 824–30.

5. Dité P, Vacek E, Stefan H, Koudelka J, Pozler O, Králová M. Endoscopic retrograde cholangiopancreatography in childhood. *Hepatogastroenterol* 1992; **39:** 291–3.

6. Brown KO, Goldschmiedt M. Endoscopic therapy of biliary and pancreatic disorders in children. *Endoscopy* 1994; **26:** 719–23.

7. Lemmel T, Hawes R, Sherman S, *et al.* Endoscopic evaluation and therapy of recurrent pancreatitis and pancreaticobiliary pain in the pediatric population. *Gastrointest Endosc* 1994; **40:** A54.

8. Guelrud M, Mujica C, Jaen D, Plaz J, Arias J. The role of ERCP in the diagnosis and treatment of idiopathic recurrent pancreatitis in children and adolescents. *Gastrointest Endosc* 1994; **40:** 428–36.

9. Pitchumoni CS. Special problems of tropical pancreatitis. *Clin Gastroenterol* 1984; **13:** 941–59.

10. Thomas PG, Augustine P, Ramesh H, *et al.* Observations and surgical management of tropical pancreatitis in Kerala and southern India. *World J Surg* 1990; **14:** 32–42.

11. Kozarek RA, Christie D, Barclay G. Endoscopic therapy of pancreatitis in the pediatric population. *Gastrointest Endosc* 1993; **39:** 665–9.

12. Stephen TC, Younoszai MK, Tyson RW, *et al.* Fibrosing pancreatitis associated with pericholangitis and cholangitis in a child. *J Pediatr Gastroenterol Nutr* 1992; **15:** 208–12.

13. Meneely RL, O'Neill JA, Gishan FK. Fibrosing pancreatitis. An obscure cause of painless obstructive jaundice: a case report and review of the literature. *Pediatrics* 1981; **67:** 136–9.

14. Wheatley MJ, Coran AG. Obstructive jaundice secondary to chronic pancreatitis in children: report of two cases and review of the literature. *Surgery* 1988; **104:** 863–9.

15. Buchta RM, Bell L. Chronic fibrosing pancreatitis in a 12-year-old female. *J Adolesc Health* 1991; **12:** 395–7.

16. Ihse I, Borch K, Larsson J. Chronic pancreatitis: results of operations for relief of pain. *World J Surg* 1990; **14:** 53–8.

17. Mettenry L, Gore DC, DeMaria FJ, Zfass AM. Endoscopic treatment of dilated-duct chronic pancreatitis with pancreatic stents: preliminary results of a sham-controlled, blinded, crossover trial to predict surgical outcome. *Am J Gastroenterol* 1993; **88:** A221.

18. Lans JI, Geenen JE, Johanson JF, Hogan WJ. Endoscopic therapy in patients with pancreas divisum and acute pancreatitis: a prospective, randomized, controlled clinical trial. *Gastrointest Endosc* 1992; **38:** 430–4.

19. Soehendra N, Grimm H, Schreiber HW. Endoskopisch-transpapillare drainage des ductus wirsungianus bei der chronischen pankreatitis, *Dtsch Med Wschr* 1986; **111:** 727–31.

20. Huibregtse K, Schneider B, Vrij AA, Tytgat GNJ. Endoscopic pancreatic drainage in chronic pancreatitis. *Gastrointest Endosc* 1988; **34:** 9–15.

21. Kozarek RA, Patterson DJ, Ball TJ, Traverso LW. Endoscopic placement of pancreatic stents and drains in the management of pancreatitis. *Ann Surg* 1989; **209:** 261–6.

22. Coleman SD, Eisen GM, Throughton AB, Cotton PB. Endoscopic treatment in pancreas divisum. *Am J Gastroenterol* 1994; **89:** 1152–5.

23. Kozarek RA. Pancreatic stents can induce ductal changes consistent with chronic pancreatitis. *Gastrointest Endosc* 1990; **36:** 93–5.

24. Gulliver DJ, Edmunds S, Baker M, *et al.* Stent placement for benign pancreatic disease: correlation between ERCP findings and clinical response. *Am J Roent* 1992; **159:** 751–5.

25. Schneider MU, Lux G. Floating pancreatic duct concrements in chronic pancreatitis. Pain relief by endoscopic removal. *Endoscopy* 1985; **17:** 8–10.

26. Fuji T, Amano H, Ohmura R *et al.* Endoscopic pancreatic sphincterotomy. Technique and evaluation. *Endoscopy* 1989; **21:** 27–30.

27. Sherman S, Lehman GA, Hawes RH, *et al.* Pancreatic ductal stones: frequency of successful endoscopic removal and improvement in symptoms. *Gastrointest Endosc* 1991; **37:** 511–7.

28. Kozarek RA, Ball TJ, Patterson DJ. Pancreatic duct stone removal in the treatment of chronic pancreatitis. *Am J Gastroenterol* 1992; **87:** 600–3.

29. Brown K, Goldschmiedt M. Use of ERCP with pancreatic and biliary sphincterotomy for treatment of familial pancreatitis in a 2 year old pediatric patient. *Gastrointest Endosc* 1993; **39:** A309.

30. Sauerbruch T, Holi J, Sackmann M, *et al.* Extracorporeal lithotripsy of pancreatic stones in patients with chronic pancreatitis and pain: a prospective follow-up study. *Gut* 1992; **33:** 969–72.

31. Delhaye M, Vandermeeren A, Baize M, *et al.* Extracorporeal shock-wave lithotripsy of pancreatic calculi. *Gastroenterology* 1992; **102:** 610–20.

32. Grimm H, Meyer H, Nam VC, Soehendra N. New modalities for treating chronic pancreatitis. *Endoscopy* 1989; **21:** 70–4.

33. Jakobs R, Maier M, Riemann JF. Laser lithotripsy of pancreatic stones: *in vitro* studies and first clinical results. *Gastrointest Endosc* 1994; **40:** A25.

34. Rösch W, Phillip J, Gebhardt Ch. Endoscopic duct obstruction in chronic pancreatitis. *Endoscopy* 1979; **11:** 43–5.

35. Rosch W. The value of endoscopic occlusion of the pancreatic duct. *Endoscopy* 1983; **15:** 175–7.

36. Bradley EL, Gonzalez AC, Clements JJr. Acute pancreatitis pseudocysts: incidence and implications. *Ann Surg* 1976; **184:** 734–7.

37. Siegleman SS. CT of fluid collections associated with pancreatitis. *Am J Radiol* 1980; **134:** 1121–5.

38. Sarles JC, Sahel J, Sarles H. Cysts and pseudocysts of the pancreas. In HT Howat, H Sarles, eds. *The exocrine pancreas.* Philodelphia: W. B. Saunders 1979; 463.

39. Yeo CT, Bastidas JA, Lynch-Nyhan A, Fishman EK, Zinner MJ, Cameron JL. The natural history of pancreatic pseudocysts documented by computer tomography. *Surg Gyneco Obstet* 1990; **170:** 411–7.

40. Bourliere M, Sarles H. Pancreatic cysts and pseudocysts associated with acute and chronic pancreatitis. *Dig Dis Sci* 1989; **34:** 343–8.

41. Beebe DS, Bubrick MP, Onstand GR, Hitchcock CR. Management of pancreatic pseudocysts. *Surg Gynecol Obstet* 1984; **159:** 562–4.

42. vanSonnenberg E, Wittich GR, Casola G, *et al.* Percutaneous drainage of infected and noninfected pancreatic pseudocysts: experience in 101 cases. *Radiology* 1989; **170:** 757–61.

43. Cremer M, Deviere J, Engelholm L. Endoscopic management of cysts and pseudocysts in chronic pancreatitis: long-term follow-up after 7 years of experience. *Gastrointest Endosc* 1989; **35:** 1–9.

44. Sahel J. Endoscopic drainage of pancreatic cysts. *Endoscopy* 1991; **23:** 181–4.

45. Smits ME, Rauws EA, Tytgat GN, Huibregtse K. The efficacy of endoscopic treatment of pancreatic pseudocysts. *Gastrointest Endosc* 1995; **42:** 202–7.

46. Dohmoto M, Rupp KD. Endoscopic drainage of pancreatic pseudocysts. *Surg Endosc* 1992; **6:** 118–24.

47. Kozarek RA, Ball TJ, Patterson DJ,Freeny PC, Ryan JA, Traverso LW. Endoscopic transpapillary therapy for disrupted pancreatic duct and peripancreatic fluid collections. *Gastroenterology* 1991; **100:** 1362–70.

48. Barthet M, Sahel J, Bodiou-Bertei CH, Bernard JP. Endoscopic transpapillary drainage of pancreatic pseudocysts. *Gastrointest Endosc* 1995; **42:** 208–13.

49. Catalano MF, Geenen JE, Schmalz MJ, Johnson GK, Dean RS, Hogan WJ. Treatment of pancreatic pseudocysts with ductal communication by transpapillary pancreatic duct endoprosthesis. *Gastrointest Endosc* 1995; **42:** 214–8.

50. Binmoeller KF, Seifert H, Walter A, Soehendra N. Transpapillary and transmural drainage of pancreatic pseudocyst. *Gastrointest Endosc* 1995; **42:** 219–24.

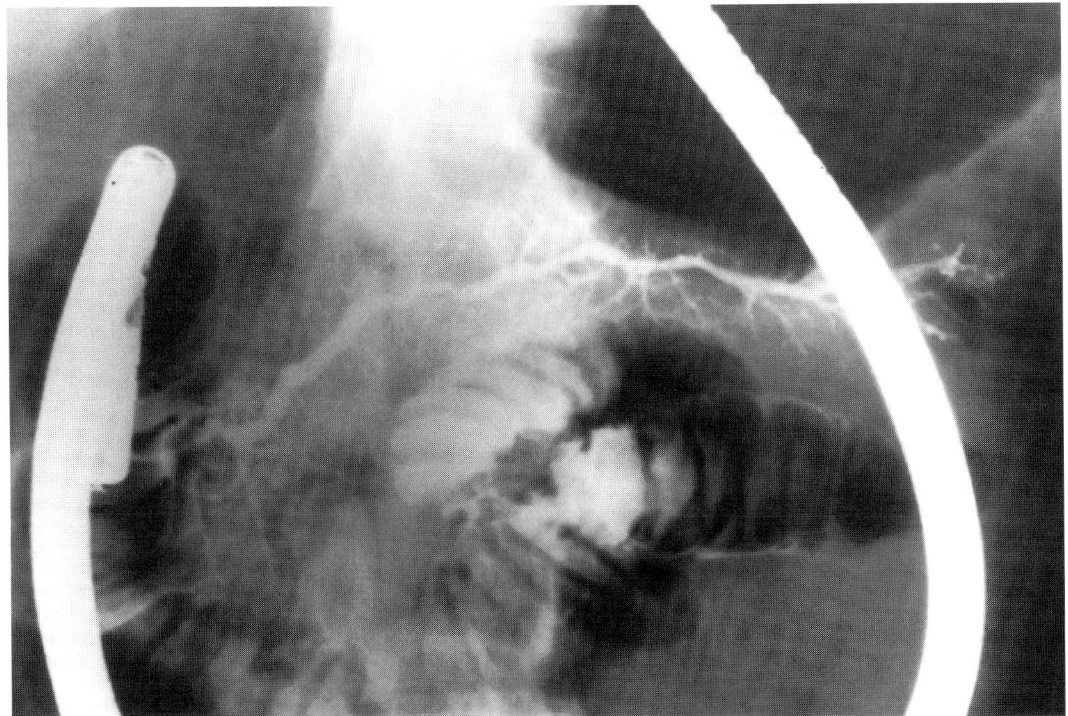

***Figure 5.1***
Chronic pancreatitis (mild changes) in a 9-year-old female. Mild dilatation of the main pancreatic duct. Dilated and irregular primary and secondary branches.

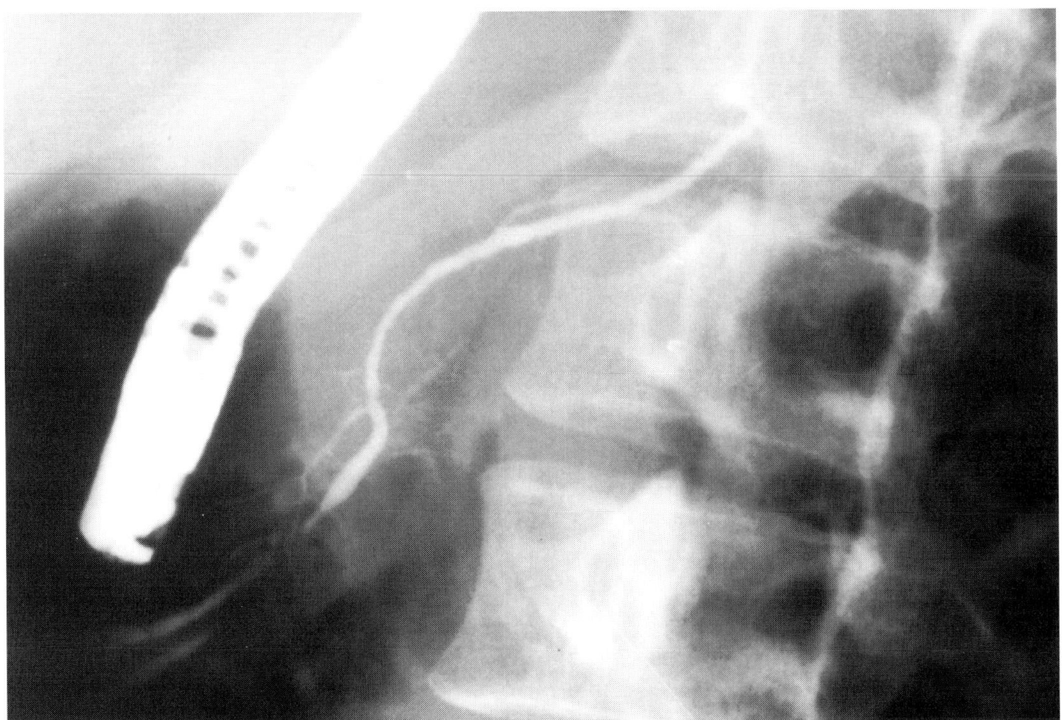

***Figure 5.2***
Chronic pancreatitis (mild changes) in a 15-year-old male. Normal caliber pancreatic duct with irregular contour.

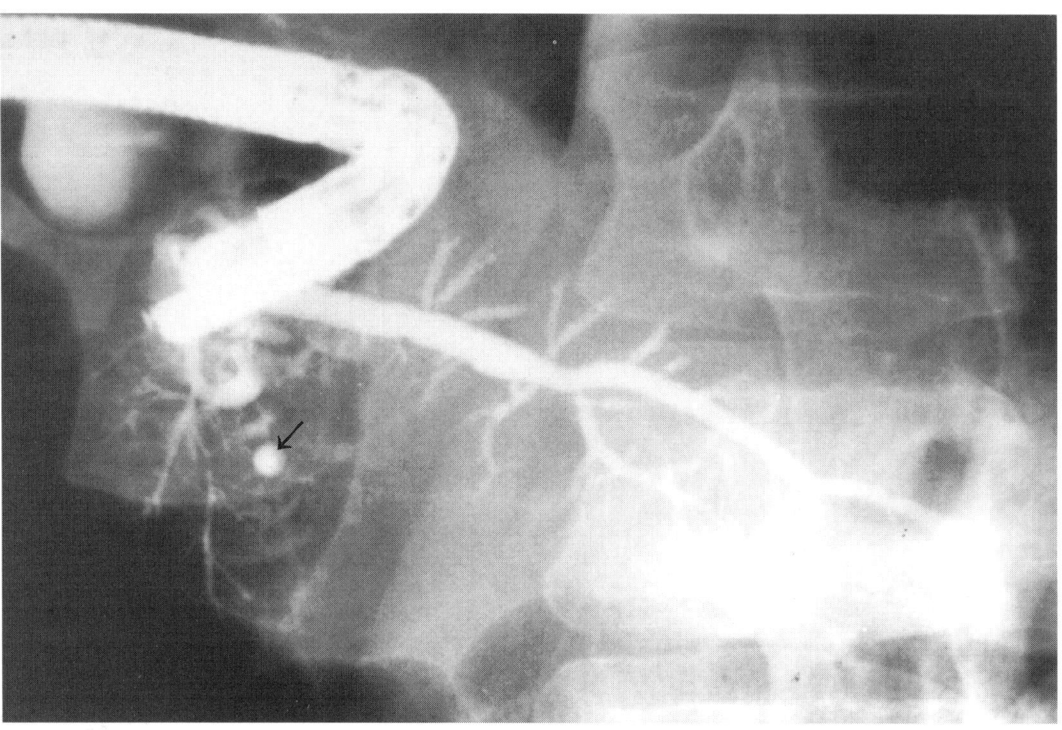

***Figure 5.3***
Chronic pancreatitis (moderate changes) in a 18-year-old male. More marked dilatation of the main pancreatic duct and primary, secondary and tertiary branches. Small pancreatic pseudocyst (↑) and pronounced acinarization.

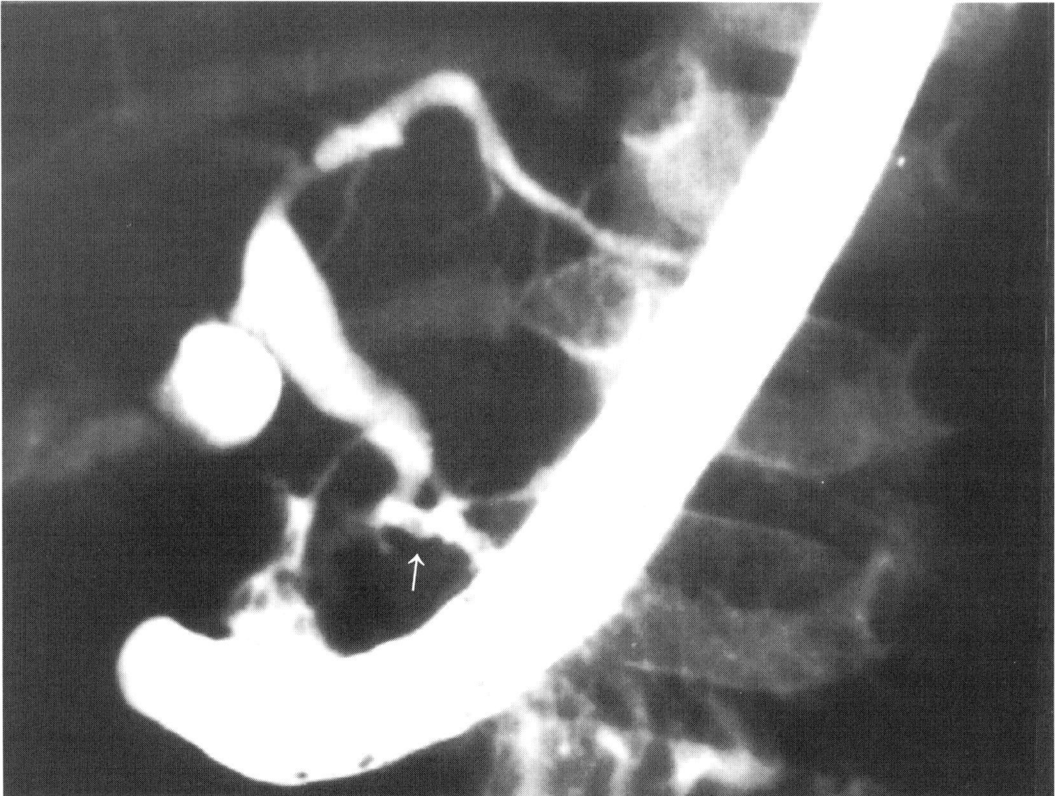

***Figure 5.4***
Chronic pancreatitis (severe changes) in a 4-year-old male. Marked dilatation of the main pancreatic duct with stones (↑). Narrow distal common bile duct probably due to chronic pancreatitis producing encasement of the bile duct.

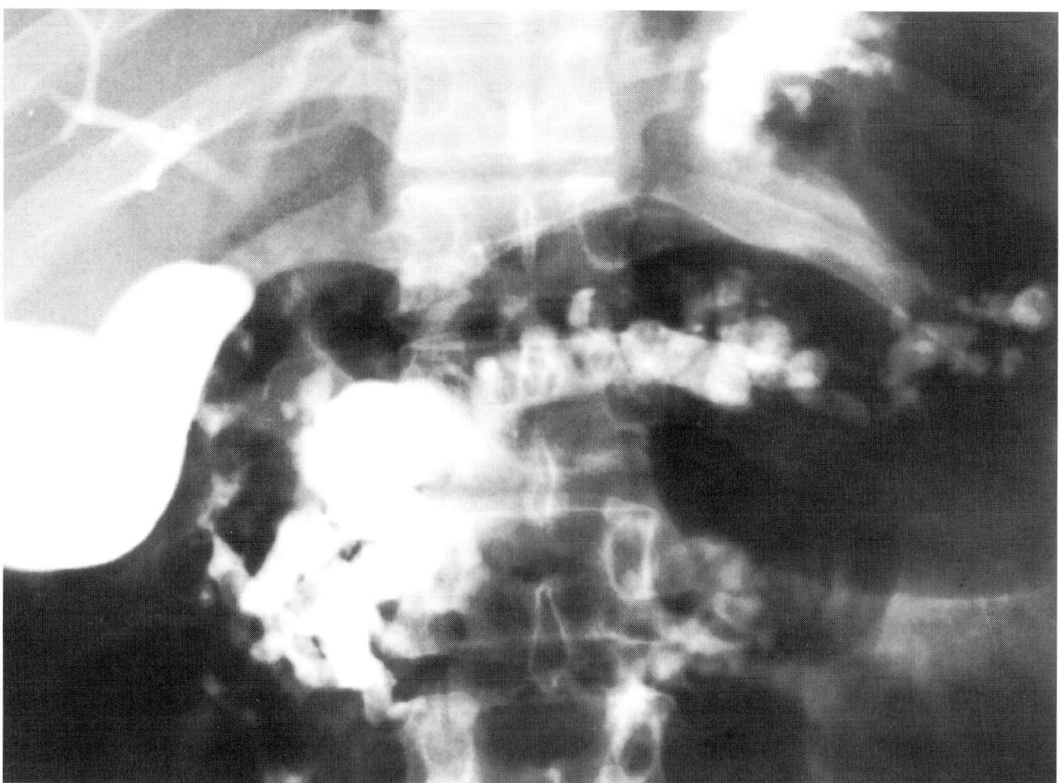

**_Figure 5.5_**
Chronic pancreatitis (severe changes) in a 6-year-old female. Marked dilatation and irregularity of the main pancreatic duct with multiple stenotic lesions and intraluminal calculi. Marked dilatation of the side branches with lacunar collections of contrast material.

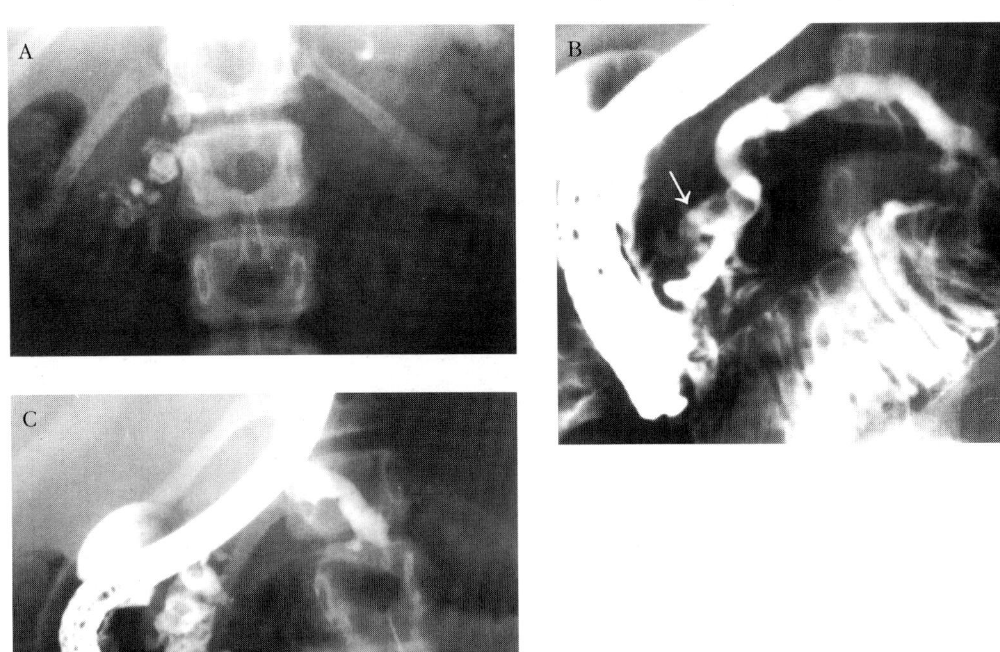

**Figure 5.6**

Juvenile tropical pancreatitis in a 6-year-old female. (A) Multiple pancreatic calcifying stones. (B) Severe pancreatic duct changes with pancreatic stones in the accessory duct (↑). A pancreatic duct sphincterotomy was performed. (C) After 1 year, the patient developed another attack of acute pancreatitis. An ERCP showed more marked dilatation of the pancreatic duct with multiple pancreatic stones. A Puestow operation was performed.

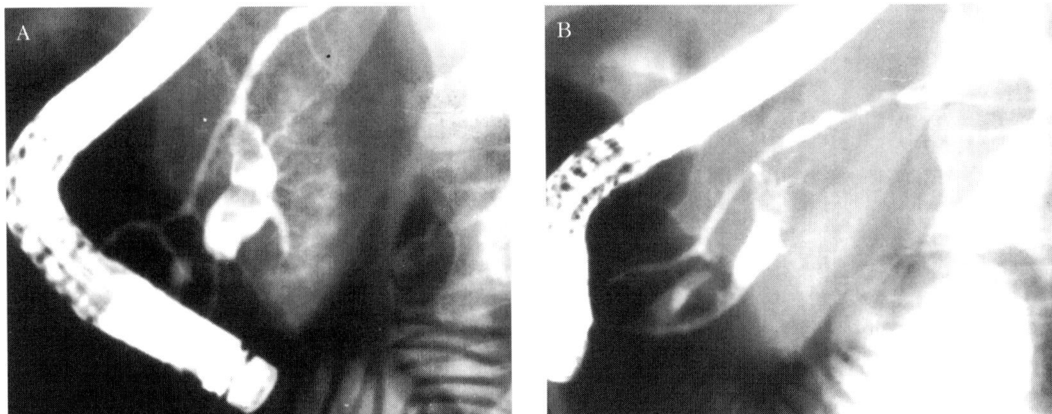

**Figure 5.7**

Chronic pancreatitis in a 19-year-old female with severe pain. (A) Severe pancreatic duct changes with multiple stones in the ventral pancreatic duct and pronounced acinarization. Moderate pancreatic changes in a dominant Santorini duct. (B) After endoscopic sphincterotomy, partial pancreatic stone extraction was performed. A wide open distal pancreatic duct can be observed. The patient remained asymptomatic for the following 18 months.

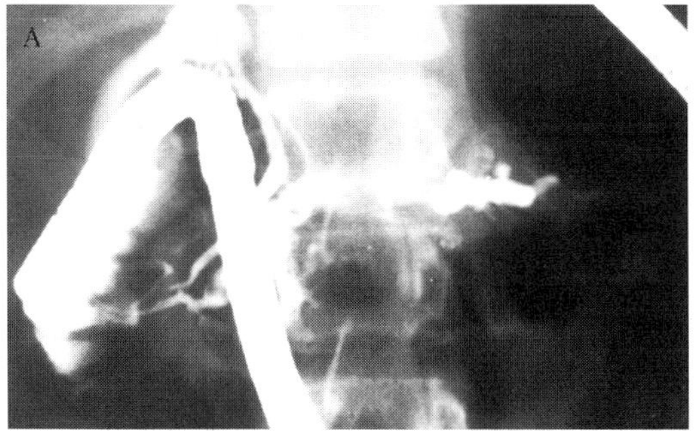

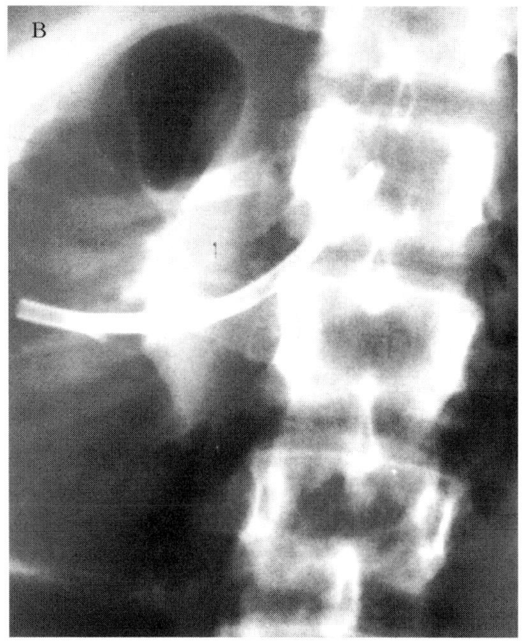

**Figure 5.8**

Hereditary chronic pancreatitis in a 12-year-old male. (A) Severe pancreatic duct changes with multiple pancreatic stones. Normal biliary tree. (B) After pancreatic sphincterotomy and stone extraction, a 10-French pancreatic stent was left in place for 30 days. The patient remained symptom free for 26 months.

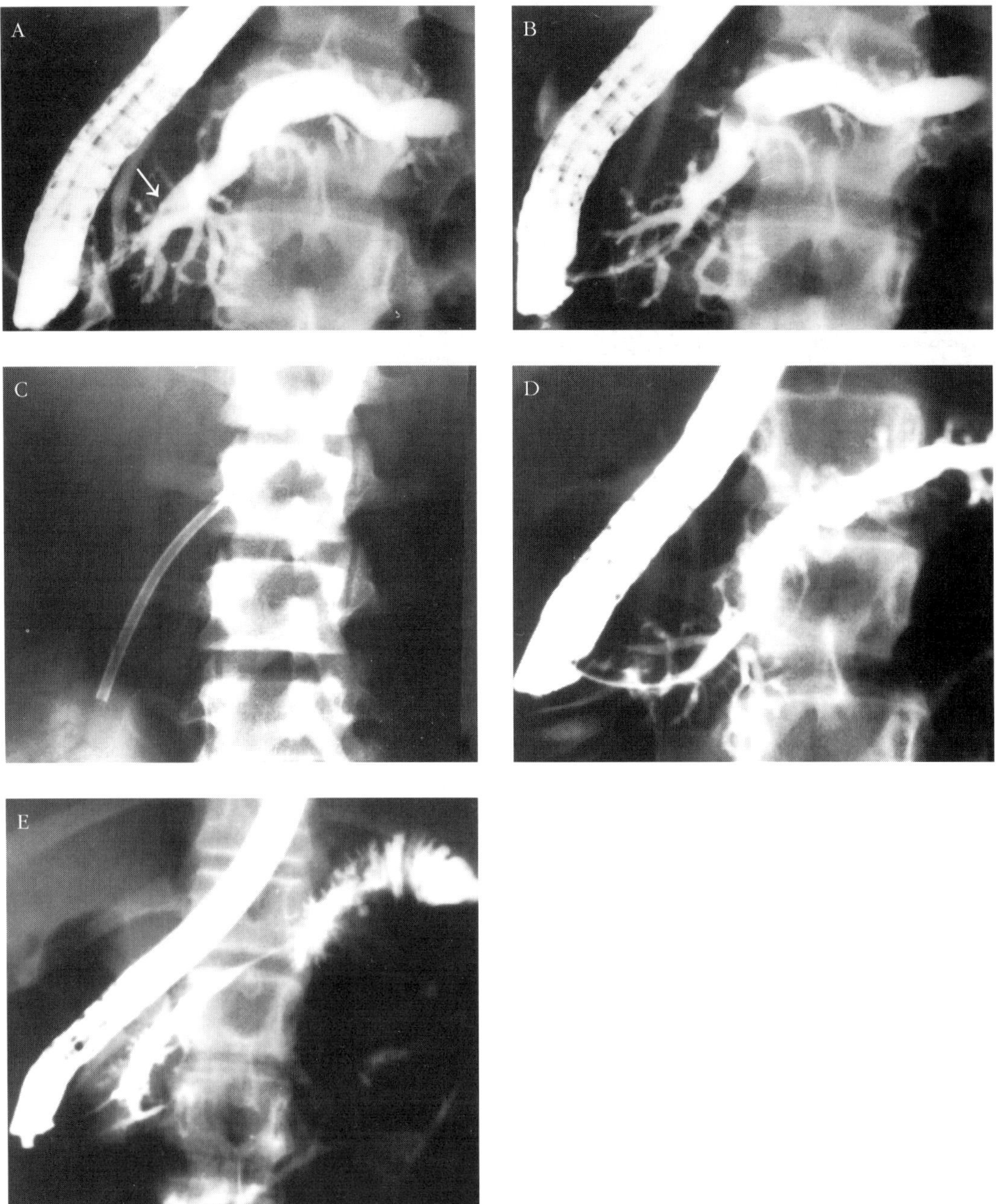

**Figure 5.9**

Juvenile tropical pancreatitis in an 8-year-old female. (A) Severe pancreatic duct changes with a stone (↑). Normal common bile duct. (B) After pancreatic sphincterotomy a Fogarty balloon was used to extract the stone. (C) A 7-French stent was left in place for 30 days. (D) After a follow-up of 12 months the pancreatic duct changes improved. After 2 years, the patient had severe pain and a Puestow operation was performed. She remained asymptomatic in the following year. (E) An ERCP showed narrowing of the distal pancreatic duct with excellent drainage to the jejunum.

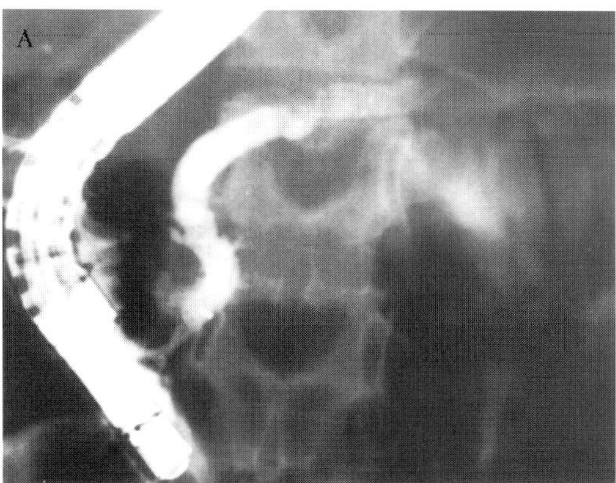
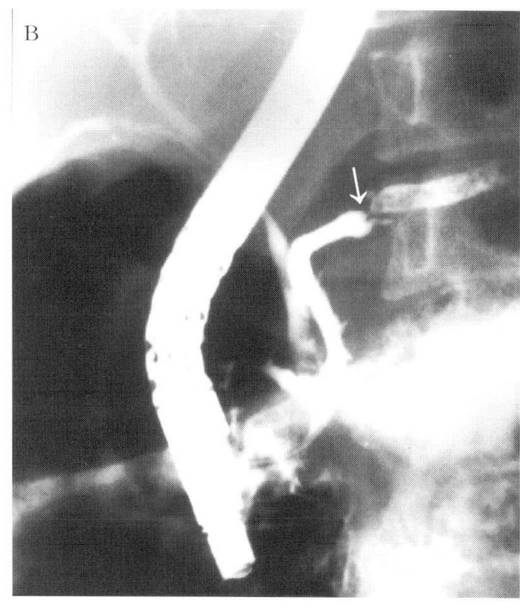

## *Figure 5.10*

Cystic fibrosis and chronic pancreatitis in a 9-year-old female with recurrent pancreatitis. (A) A pancreatogram showing dilated main pancreatic duct and blunted side branches with multiple stones. A pancreatic sphincterotomy with stone extraction was performed. (B) After 1½ years, the patient had two attacks of acute pancreatitis. A pancreatogram demonstrated a dilated pancreatic duct without stones at the head of the pancreas. A narrow stricture at the body of the pancreas (↑) with multiple prestenotic stones was visualized. A Puestow operation was performed.

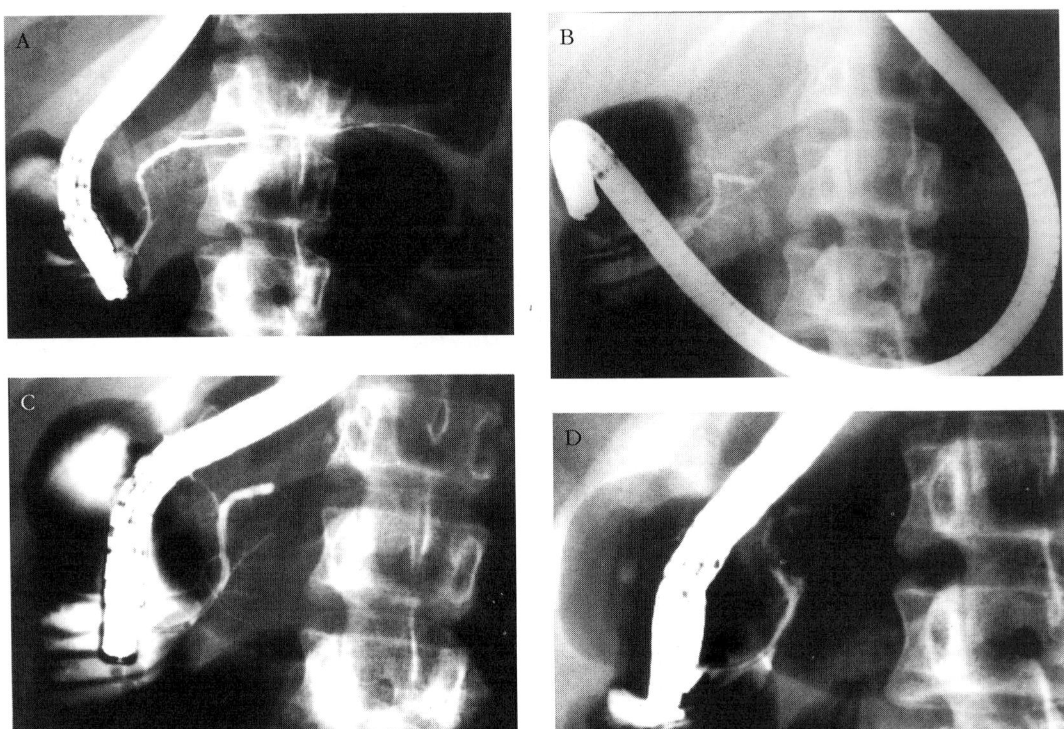

**_Figure 5.11_**

Chronic pancreatitis treated by occlusion of the pancreatic duct with cyanocrilate glue in a 18-year-old female with intractable pain and narcotic addiction. (A) A narrow and irregular pancreatic duct. The patient was treated surgically by subtotal pancreatectomy without clinical improvement. (B) Eight months after surgery, a normal caliber pancreatic duct with acinarization was visualized at the head of the pancreas. Two milliliters of cyanocrilate glue was injected in the pancreatic duct. The patient remained symptom free during 2 years. (C) An ERCP performed after 1 year of cyanoacrilate injection showed a dilated pancreatic duct with filling of primary and secondary branches without acinarization. (D) After 2 years, the patient developed severe chronic pain and a second cyanocrilate injection was performed. An ERCP performed before cyanoacrilate injection, showed the pancreatic duct with opacification of the accessory duct and a "Santorinicele". She remained asymptomatic for the ensuing 3 years.

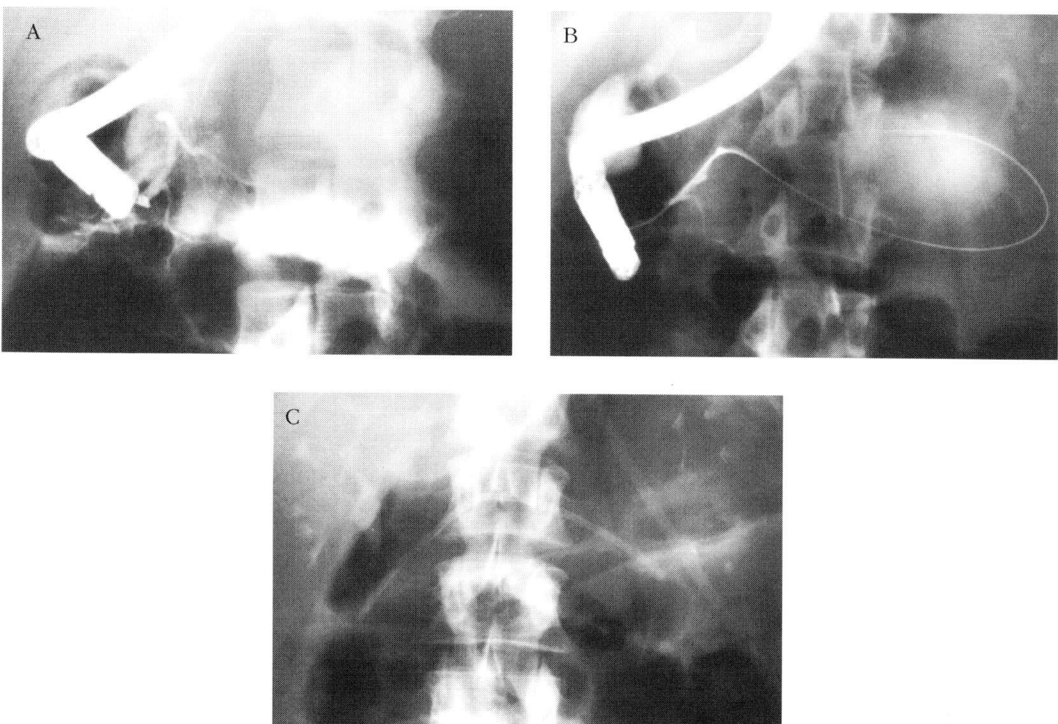

**Figure 5.12**

Pancreatic pseudocyst with ductal communication treated by transpapillary pancreatic duct endoprosthesis in a 13-year-old female. (A) Pancreatogram demonstrating partial filling of a pseudocyst in the body and tail of the pancreas. (B) After endoscopic sphincterotomy of the pancreatic and biliary sphincters a guidewire is introduced into the cystic cavity. (C) A 7F endoprosthesis is placed beyond the stricture.

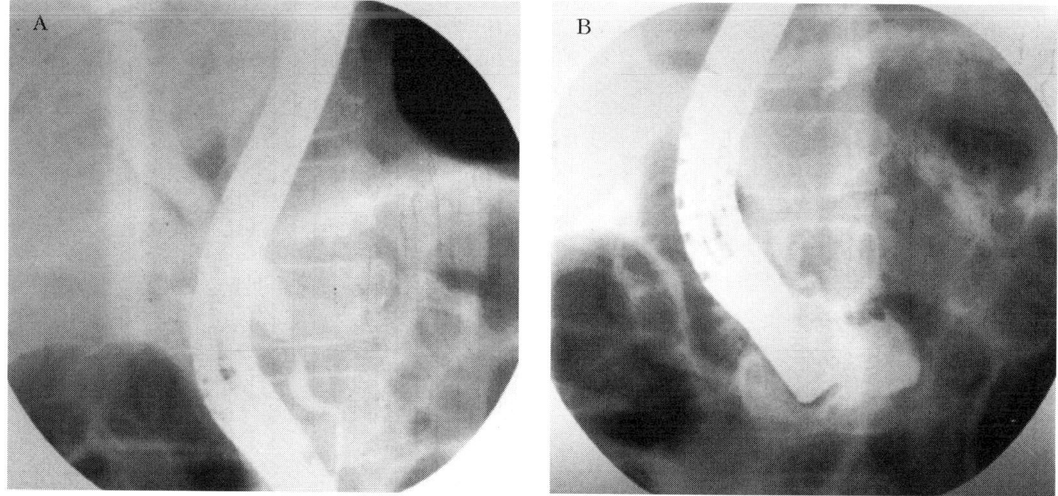

**Figure 5.13**

Double duct sign due to chronic fibrosing pancreatitis in an 8-year-old girl presenting with obstructive jaundice. (A) Stricture of the intrapancreatic portion of the distal common bile duct. (B) Pancreatogram shows long stricture in head of pancreas and irregular and mildly dilated duct upstream in body of pancreas.

# CHAPTER 6

# Pancreatic trauma

Pancreatic trauma occurs frequently in childhood as a result of bicycle and a variety of other accidents. In adolescents and young adults, motorcycle accidents are common causes (1). Pancreatic trauma may lead to pancreatitis and pancreatic ductal rupture which can be asymptomatic for the first few days (2). The pancreas is positioned over the spine, hence its location lends the organ vulnerable to injury by blunt abdominal trauma which may fracture or sever the ducts. Traumatic pancreatitis and its sequelae have significant morbidity and mortality (3,4) and diagnosis with subsequent therapy should be accomplished as soon as possible to improve outcome (5). Abdominal ultrasound and spiral CT scanning are excellent methods of evaluating the pancreas (6) but it cannot determine the integrity of the pancreatic duct. Barkin *et al.* found that none of 12 patients who underwent abdominal CT had abnormalities indicative of pancreatic rupture, yet three had ductal rupture (7). ERCP is diagnostic for pancreatic duct laceration showing extravasation of contrast at the point of disruption (9,10). The sensitivity and specificity of ERCP was found to be 100% for pancreatic duct disruption, whereas no combination of serum amylase, CT and peritoneal lavage was equally effective. Neither the presence of hyperamylasemia nor the peak level separated patients with fractured pancreatic duct (4).

Hall *et al.* reported four cases of pancreatic trauma in children aged 2–13 years and recommended early ERCP to identify the presence and location of duct leakage for patients requiring urgent surgery (9). Similar results have been found by Rescorla *et al.* (10) who performed ERCP in 6 children aged 2½ to 8 years after pancreatic trauma. Patients with normal ductograms are treated conservatively. Patients with duct disruption may be managed surgically or by transpapillary stenting. The site of duct disruption can be bridged by wire-guided stent (11). Traumatic pancreatitis may result in pseudocyst formation and in extrinsic compression of the distal common bile duct resulting in obstructive jaundice. This may be successfully managed endoscopically by temporary biliary endoprostheses (Fig. 6.1).

## References


1. Yellin AE, Vecchione TR, Donovan AJ. Distal pancreatectomy for pancreatic trauma. *Am J Surg* 1972; **124:** 135–41.
2. Northrup W, Simmons RL. Pancreatic trauma: a review. *Surgery* 1972, **71:** 27–43.
3. Vane DW, Grosfeld JL, West KW, Rescorla FJ. Pancreatic disorders in infancy and childhood: experience with 92 cases. *J Pediatr Surg* 1989; **24:** 771–6.
4. Taxier M, Sivak MV, Cooperman AM, Sullivan BH. Endoscopic retrograde pancreatography in the evaluation of trauma to the pancreas. *Surg Gynecol Obstet* 1980; **150:** 65–8.
5. Whittwell AE, Gomez GA, Byers P, Kreis DJ, Manten H, Casillas VJ. Blunt pancreatic trauma: prospective evaluation of early endoscopic retrograde pancreatography. *S Med J* 1989; **82:** 586–91.

6. Federle MP, Crass RA, Jeffrey RB, Trunkey DD. Computed tomography in blunt abdominal trauma. *Arch Surg* 1982; **117:** 645–50.

7. Barkin JS, Ferstenberg RM, Panullo W, Manten HD, Davis RC. Endoscopic retrograde cholangiopancreatography in pancreatic trauma. *Gastrointest Endosc* 1988, **34:** 102–5.

8. Bozymski EM, Orlando RC, Holt JW. Traumatic disruption of the pancreatic duct demonstrated by endoscopic retrograde pancreatography. *J Trauma* 1981; **21:** 244–5.

9. Hall RI, Lavelle MI, Venables CW. Use of ERCP to identify the site of traumatic injuries of the main pancreatic duct in children. *Br J Surg* 1986; **73:** 411–2.

10. Rescorla FJ, Plumley DA, Sherman S, *et al.* The efficacy of early ERCP in pediatric pancreatic trauma. *J Pediatr Surg* 1995; **30:** 336–40.

11. Kozarek RA, Ball TJ, Patterson DJ, Freeny PC, Ryan JA, Traverso W. Endoscopic transpapillary therapy for disrupted pancreatic duct and peripancreatic fluid collections. *Gastroenterology* 1991; **100:** 1362–70.

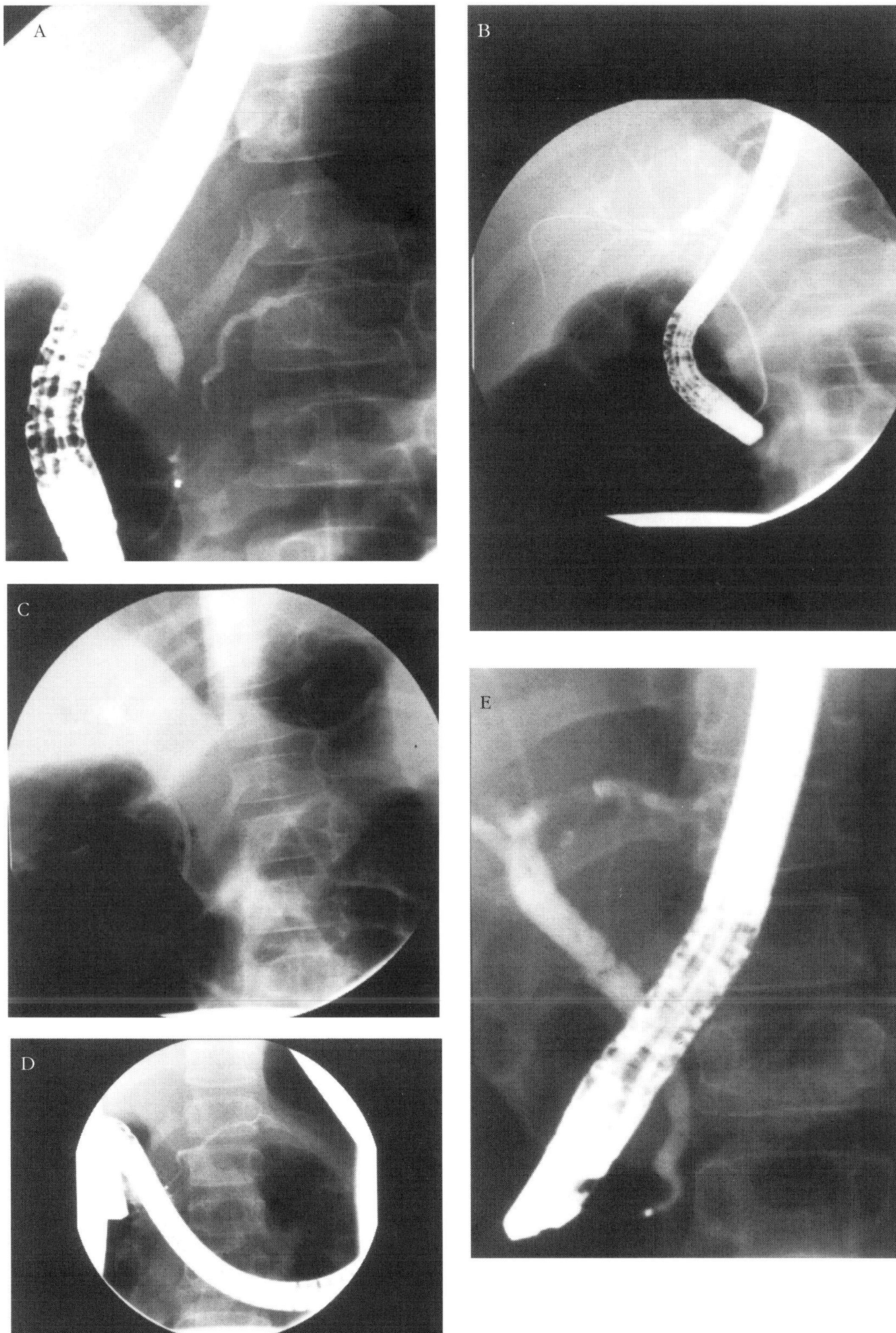

**Figure 6.1**

(A) ERCP radiograph showing distal bile duct stricture and corresponding narrowing of the pancreatic duct in the head of the pancreas in a 9-year-old patient with post-traumatic pancreatitis. (B) Insertion of endoscopic biliary endoprostheses for the relief of biliary obstruction. (C) Position of biliary endoprostheses immediately after placement. (D) ERP 3 months later showing resolution of the ductal stenosis. (E) ERC 3 months after stent placement with complete resolution of distal bile duct stricture and after removal of endoprosthesis, patient has remained well and asymptomatic.